Endorsements

"Lou Ignarro is a quite simply, a living legend — one of the great Nobel Laureates whose lifework has advanced human knowledge about health and disease. Being acquainted with a Nobel Laureate is a rarity for almost anyone, but I've known Lou for almost two decades. He is not only brilliant and accomplished, but a passionate and engaging storyteller who can make anyone feel like they understand who he is as a person, how he came to make the scientific discoveries that led to his Nobel Prize, and how these discoveries relate to them. Nitric oxide (NO) is one of the body's great health signals, and much of what we know about it today emanated from Louis Ignarro (including the development of Viagra). This book is Lou's memoir, and in it, he elegantly tells the story of his life, starting from his humble beginning as the child of uneducated immigrant parents from Italy, building sandcastles on a New York beach, to his boyhood interests in chemistry and making explosives, to his groundbreaking discoveries about nitric oxide. This is a unique window into how an ordinary man overcame hardships to make extraordinary contributions to the world as a scientist. He also gives a rare first-person view of the Stockholm Concert Hall where the King of Sweden presented him with the 1998 Nobel Prize in Medicine or Physiology. Throughout this fascinating book, you also discover that Lou's story is connected with that of Alfred Nobel, the man who established the Prize itself!"

— *William Li, MD. President of the*
Angiogenesis Foundation, Boston

"The son of uneducated immigrant parents from Italy, Lou Ignarro climbed to the top of his profession, for which he was awarded the Nobel Prize in Medicine. In this book, Lou elegantly describes the hardships he had to overcome in every step of his journey. A good read."

— *Andrew Weil, MD, PhD. Director of the Arizona Center*
for Integrative Medicine at the University of Arizona

"Lou Ignarro's transfixing, riveting, true story takes you through a Horatio Alger tale as the son of immigrant parents in Brooklyn to a Nobel Prize in Medicine in Stockholm. The story reveals an uncanny parallel between Lou's life and that of Alfred Nobel himself, for whom the Prize is named – both experimenting with the chemistry of "nitro" compounds – in the case of Nobel, harnessing these compounds as the explosive dynamite, and for Ignarro discovering nitroglycerin-like compounds function in the human body as vasodilators. The one difference – Lou doesn't blow up his laboratory!"

— Stuart Lipton, MD, PhD. Professor & Director, Neurosciences Translational Center, Department of Molecular Medicine, The Scripps Research Institute, La Jolla

"This elegantly written true story is a must-read for anyone wanting to understand the making of a Nobel laureate in Medicine, from early childhood to the awards ceremony in Stockholm. Moreover, Lou Ignarro gets very personal and reveals much about himself and his upbringing. He was the one key person to help me change the world of newborn pediatric medicine by saving thousands of newborns, turning blue babies pink."

— Warren Zapol, MD, Professor and Chairman, Dept. of Anesthesia, Massachusetts General Hospital

"Lou Ignarro elegantly describes the uphill and circuitous path taken from building sand castles on the beach in New York to receiving the Nobel Prize from the King of Sweden."

— Sir Richard Roberts, PhD, biochemist and molecular biologist, New England Biolabs, Nobel Prize in Physiology or Medicine (1993)

"Lou Ignarro has written a compelling autobiography describing how his lifelong pursuit of scientific discovery resulted in winning the Nobel Prize in Medicine. By following his scientific curiosity, this son of Italian immigrants in New York became both a world-renowned scientist and a great educator. This true story of the life of a Nobel laureate is inspirational."

— Richard van Breemen, PhD, Endowed Chair and Director of Linus Pauling Institute, Oregon State University

Dr. NO

Dr. NO

Dr. NO

The Discovery That Led
to a Nobel Prize & Viagra

Louis J. Ignarro, PhD

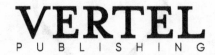

Dr. NO

Copyright © 2021 by Louis J. Ignarro, PhD

For information, contact Vertel Publishing at
2837 Rivers Avenue
Charleston, South Carolina 29405

First edition

Manufactured in the United States of America

1 3 5 7 9 10 8 6 4 3

Hardcover ISBN: 978-1-64112-029-6
Paperback ISBN: 978-1-64112-032-6
eBook ISBN: 978-1-64112-030-2

Library of Congress Cataloging-in-Publication Data has been applied for.

This book is dedicated to the two strongest women in my life- my wife and partner, Dr. Sharon Williams Ignarro, and my mother, Frances Ignarro. Sharon has been my strongest supporter through all the ups and downs of this wild ride in completing my book. She has been my inspiration for healthy living and my enthusiastic coach in all of our athletic endeavors. My mom was by my side for every step of my journey to the pinnacle of scientific research, from dealing with my childhood explosive chemistry experiments to providing motivation to continue my basic research career in medicine. My life has been forever changed by them.

Table of Contents

PART IV: The Nobel Prize 217

"Life is either a daring adventure or nothing at all."
— *Helen Keller*

PART V: Post-Nobel and New Findings. 275

"Logic will get you from point A to point B, but imagination
will take you everywhere."
— Albert Einstein

Author's Note

This book is a memoir of my roller coaster ride from building sandcastles on the beach as a small child to receiving the Nobel Prize from the hands of His Majesty King Carl Gustaf of Sweden in 1998.

I discovered science early in life, and my passion for it never waned, steadily growing through my education at Columbia College and the University of Minnesota. I entered the professional world as a basic biomedical researcher in chemical pharmacology. I spent my research career trying to understand the causes, prevention, and treatment of inflammation and cardiovascular disease.

Early on, I learned that one requires "thick skin" to engage successfully in basic research. Along the way, there are often more downs than ups and an equal number of curveballs and fastballs. Survival depends on motivation, perseverance, and the will to "never give up." Success depends on the ability to "think outside the box." Discovery depends on getting up every time I fell and leaving a clear trail behind me.

This isn't just a scientist's story; it's an American story. Only in America can the child of uneducated Italian immigrants start out a struggling student, barely able to speak English, and go on to win the Nobel Prize.

Though I detail my scientific experiments and discoveries, this is ultimately a story of perseverance, teamwork, and awe—there's even a couple of love stories. My wish is that as you read this, you will learn not only an intimate view of my path to discovery but also the inspiration and simplicity of science. My greatest hope is that my story will inspire tomorrow's scientists to see how they might carve their own path from a beginner's chemistry set to winning the Nobel Prize.

Foreword

The discovery of Nitric Oxide and its role in the health of the cardiovascular system is an exciting story of the vision and energy of Dr. Lou Ignarro, who rose from humble beginnings to ultimately win the Nobel Prize in Physiology or Medicine in 1998. The finding that nitric oxide, or NO gas, had a role in human physiology was proven by Dr. Ignarro through a series of carefully designed studies, first at Tulane University Medical Center and then at UCLA School of Medicine. Through collaboration with a group of distinguished investigators including other Nobel Prize winners over the span of his career, the details of NO's discovery demonstrate how science is advanced by working collaboratively with a community of scientists with diverse expertise. The myth of the lone scientist in the laboratory is no longer possible given the complexity of biomedical research. Still, that observation does not minimize the contributions of the seminal and visionary work of Dr. Lou Ignarro that led to the discovery of a new neurotransmitter that was a gas, which no one believed existed in human cells. Louis Pasteur famously stated that "chance the prepared mind".

This is certainly the case in the relationship of NO to the invention of drugs like Viagra for erectile dysfunction.

If you are a junior scientist, a young person who aspires to have a scientific career or have an enquiring mind, you will appreciate the rigor of his research strategies over many years and several institutions. He demonstrated for the first time, to the surprise of many, that a gas made of two atoms could be a messenger molecule of immense significance in the body. He had the creative vision that nitric oxide is produced whenever the nervous system is stimulated to increase blood flow and supply oxygen and nutrients to your body's cells. Dr. Ignarro gathered the specialized technology to prove that nitric oxide is made in the single layer of endothelial cells lining the arteries of all the organs of the body.

In this book, you will get an intimate view of Dr. Ignarro's personality, tremendous creative energy, vision, imagination, courage, struggles, and triumphs over the course of his life. You will be taken on an intimate journey of his thoughts and dreams starting from his early childhood interest in chemistry, which resulted in some accidental explosive results, to his ultimate focus on the detailed pharmacology of nitric oxide's production and action in cardiovascular health and disease. You will be taken on a detailed journey through the laboratory experiments that proved the importance of NO in relaxing blood vessels to increase blood flow, as well as the collaborations and insights from the work of other scientists that led to the discovery of the role of NO in cardiovascular health and erectile dysfunction. In the process, you will meet many prominent scientists who contributed to Dr. Ignarro's journey of discovery. You will experience the thrill of the Nobel Prize award ceremony in Stockholm and the aftermath of the adulation and celebration that followed for Dr. Ignarro.

I have been honored to write these words introducing this amazing story of my friend and colleague, Dr. Lou Ignarro, who is a warm human being who loves Italian cuisine, red wine, model trains, and family. We have many areas of parallel and intersecting interests in medicine, physiology, nutrition, and exercise. The basic and clinical laboratories of the UCLA Center for Human Nutrition continue the work begun by Dr. Ignarro on NO by studying the impact of antioxidant nutrients from fruits and vegetables and the amino acids arginine and citrulline in basic and human clinical research on blood flow and blood vessel health. A new generation of researchers will carry this work into the future, and this book should be an inspiration to them.

— David Heber, M.D., Ph.D., Founding Director, UCLA Center for Human Nutrition, author of *Primary Care Nutrition, The L.A. Shape Diet, What Color Is Your Diet?* and *Natural Remedies for a Healthy Heart* journey of discovery. You will experience the thrill of the Nobel Prize award ceremony in Stockholm, and the aftermath of the audition and celebration that followed for Dr. Ignarro.

I have been honored to write these words, introducing the amazing story of my friend and colleague, Dr. Louis Ignarro, who in turn has become one who loves to think, cure, cancer, and wine, model trains, and family. We have many areas of mutual and intersecting interests in medicine, physiology, nutrition, and exercise. The basic and clinical laboratories of the UCLA Center for Human Nutrition continue the work begun by Dr. Ignarro in NO by studying the impact of antioxidant nutrients from fruits and vegetables and the amino acid arginine and citrulline in basic and human clinical research on blood flow and blood vessel health. A new generation of researchers will carry this work into the future, and this book should be an inspiration to them.

David Heber, M.D., Ph.D., Founding Director, UCLA Center For Human Nutrition, author of Nutrition: The L.A. Shape Diet, What Color Is Your Diet and Natural Remedies for a Healthy Heart

Prologue

O ctober 12, 1998, began with my attending a scientific advisory board meeting for a small biotech company in Nice, France. The name of the company was Nicox, and it focused on developing novel anti-inflammatory drugs that worked by releasing nitric oxide (NO) selectively at sites of inflammation. I had been attending these meetings in Nice for several years and always enjoyed both the scientific discussions and the frequent walks along the beautiful sandy beaches one block away. I could never get enough of the south of France. And so, today was no different from any of my prior visits. Or was it?

Gazing out the window on a beautiful sunny morning, in the final meeting of the three-day conference, I began to daydream and, for no discernible reason, felt exceptionally content. I was so relaxed and peaceful that I dozed off for a moment. I promptly caught myself and sat up in my chair as if nothing had happened. Luckily, it seemed no one had noticed. Nevertheless, something was different about today, but I couldn't figure out what.

After the meeting ended, we all wished each other a safe trip back home, and I went for a brief stroll on the boardwalk along the beach. Walking along the beach in Nice brought back fond memories of my childhood days in Long Beach.

Once again, I felt an unusual aura of serenity, but I couldn't understand why. Perhaps, it was because I was about to catch my flight to Naples, Italy, the birthplace of my father. At the invitation of one of my scientific colleagues at the University of Napoli, I was to give a lecture on my research involving nitric oxide. I was always thrilled to visit Naples because it reminded me of Dad. I attributed my unusual calm to this upcoming trip.

One of the company drivers took me to the Côte d'Azur Airport in Nice, and I proceeded to collect my boarding pass and walk over to my departure gate, Porte A4. A few people were waiting in line, and I joined the queue. About ten minutes later, an airport attendant walked over to the gate and, picking up a microphone from the desk, said, "Is there a Professor Ignarro here at the gate?"

I responded, "Yes, I am Professor Ignarro, over here!"

The young lady rushed over to me and handed me her mobile phone. "You have an urgent telephone call from Los Angeles."

My mouth dropped open. I thought something terrible must have happened at home. The attendant told me to hurry up with the call because we had only a minute or so before boarding.

Despite all the static in the line, I asked who was calling. It turned out to be one of my close physician colleagues at UCLA. I immediately asked him if everything was okay with my laboratory and family. He responded, "Yes, all is good here. I'm calling to see how you feel ..." But I could not understand the rest of what he said because his voice was breaking up.

Finally, I was able to comprehend: "Lou, I'm just calling to congratulate you!"

"Congratulate me for what?"

"Lou, you mean to tell me that you've not heard yet?"

"Heard what?" I said in a loud, almost angry tone of voice.

"You've been awarded the Nobel Prize in Medicine!"

Precisely at that moment, the attendant yanked the phone from my hand. "So sorry, but we must board the flight now."

Bewildered and disoriented, I boarded my flight for Naples. It took only a few moments to reach my seat, but along the way, a million thoughts raced through my mind.

Was I really awarded the Nobel Prize? Me? Did I share it with anyone else? Was the prize for my work on nitric oxide? Was it for my neuroscience studies that led to the development and marketing of Viagra? What was it for?

As the plane departed, I sat back in my seat but could not relax one bit. The flight was only forty minutes, and I would, undoubtedly, find out one way or another when I landed in Naples. But the flight felt more like four hours. In attempting to put my thoughts together, I vaguely recalled that the Nobel Prizes were announced early in October at about noon. Today was October 12, and the plane had departed at noon. *Okay, maybe*, I thought.

The plane approached Capodichino Airport in Naples and landed smoothly. As we taxied to the gate, I looked out my window and saw hundreds of people on the tarmac, waiting for the plane to pull up and park.

"Oh my God!" I said out loud. "It's true!"

PART I:
The Early Years

"The only impossible journey is the one you never begin."
— *Tony Robbins*

Chapter 1:
My Early Childhood and Fascination with Science

I almost wasn't born. My father, Giacomo Ignarro, was born and raised in a coastal suburb of Naples. A carpenter and ship-builder by trade, during World War I, he and his brother Giuseppe enlisted in the Italian Navy. According to my dad, their ship was struck by a German torpedo in the mid-Atlantic and wound up docking in New York Harbor for battleship repairs.

He quickly recognized that the repairs had not been performed according to code, and having little faith that the ship would make the journey, my dad and his brother decided not to go back to Italy. They hid in the Catskill Mountains in New York until the war was over and all was forgiven by the Italian government. He later learned that the battleship never made it back to Italy. The entire crew had perished at sea.

Both my parents were born in Italy: my dad in Torre del Greco, and my mom, Francesca Russo, in Panarea, one of the tiny Aeolian Islands just off the northern coast of Sicily. Panarea is so small that one could row a boat around the entire island in only a few hours. The island had no cars, buses, trucks, or rail transportation of any kind. Except for an occasional horse and buggy, all transportation around the island was by foot. Today, Panarea is basically the same except a few roads have been built to accommodate small motor vehicles for commercial purposes.

Francesca's father (my maternal grandfather) moved his wife and five children to New York City when my mom was sixteen years old. Though they intended to eventually relocate to Los Angeles, New York would provide a waypoint to raise funds for the cross-country trip.

When my mom arrived in New York, she marveled over the sights and sounds of cars, motorbikes, trucks, and trains—none of which she had ever seen before. Mom always told me that her first sight of airplanes flying above New York, carrying people from one city to another, was "truly amazing."

About three years after Mom's arrival in New York, she met my dad-to-be for the first time, and they started to date, of sorts. Of course, this involved the two of them going to the movie house or dinner or for a walk, with brothers and sisters tagging along. That's the way it was back then in the 1930s.

As their relationship grew stronger, her father announced that he had raised sufficient funds to move the entire family to Los Angeles. Francesca, however, was not about to move away from her boyfriend. After considerable infighting and negotiating, she was allowed to remain in New York but only if she married Giacomo.

The wedding was a large, formal church affair in Brooklyn, followed by a typical Italian reception with home-cooked dishes, baked goods, wine and beer, and lots of Italian music and dancing. Giacomo was a talented operatic tenor, and he sang many Neapolitan folk tunes at the reception.

I was born about two years later in 1941, and my brother, Angelo, followed in 1944. Since the wedding, my dad became a successful carpenter and homebuilder in Long Beach, about twenty miles east of New York City. Dad was a highly skilled cabinetmaker and furnituremaker, but he mainly earned his living doing larger projects. In addition to his ability to design, plan, and build entire homes in the neighborhood, he also was hired by the city to rebuild the boardwalk—a three-mile stretch of a fifty-foot-wide wooden walkway built on top of steel and concrete pillars.

Being Italian, my parents were excellent chefs (one step above cooks), and my dad insisted on healthy Italian meals every single day of the week. Growing up, my brother and I reaped the benefits of their unique blend of Neapolitan and Sicilian cooking styles. Our home was the neighborhood's favorite place to visit for lunch or dinner.

Mom's meat sauce was indescribably delicious. Starting soon after their marriage, Mom and Dad had worked together in the kitchen for years, perfecting the meat sauce to everyone's satisfaction. My brother and I were the guinea pigs during this long series of culinary experiments. Two full days were required to prepare this special meat sauce, which imparted an incredible and unmistakable aroma throughout the house that lasted for days.

My dad was also an avid fisherman, frequently going to the ocean or bay, located on the north side of Long Beach, to fish for clams, crabs, mussels, eel, and small fish. Dad did most of the cooking when seafood was involved. He'd gotten a great deal of experience as a teenager in Naples and also had served as a cook in the Italian Navy.

Angelo and I considered ourselves fortunate to live in a family with a passion for incredible homemade cooking. Not only were the Italian meals tasty, but they also were quite healthy. My father had always forbidden the use of packaged or processed foods in our home. Everything that would eventually find its way into our mouths had to be natural and fresh. Dad even managed to make his own red wine rather than buying it from the local wine shop. Mom and Dad were special, and cooking this way every evening helped to bond our family together. According to my dad, our evening dinner was the most important time of the day.

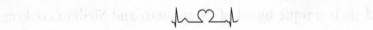

The trouble began when I was due to begin kindergarten. My teacher noted that I spoke in broken English with a distinct Italian accent. After meeting with my parents, the teacher understood the problem. My dad spoke no English, while Mom spoke English poorly. My parents were informed that I would likely have a significant learning problem unless I developed the skills to communicate properly and efficiently in English.

Upon hearing that, my mom stopped speaking Italian at home and worked hard to improve her English language skills. Dad experienced more difficulty, but he managed to learn to understand and speak some English; however, he never learned to write in it.

My first three years in grade school were arduous, not only because of the language barrier but also because neither Mom nor Dad could help me with any kind of homework. Still, my education was a priority for them. They provided me lots of motivation and inspiration and even hired tutors to work with me when I needed help.

I also received helpful support from the community. Most of my friends' parents were lawyers, doctors, engineers, tax accountants, and teachers. They were also my dad's clients. They all loved his carpentry, so someone was always nearby who was happy to give me a helping hand whenever I needed it. One of our closest neighbors was a mathematician named Mr. Kirsch, and he met with me once or twice a week to strengthen my skills and help keep me one step ahead of the class. He had the patience to listen to my nagging questions about the universe and other scientific matters. I learned later on from my mom that Mr. Kirsch was impressed with my interest in science. He told her that he knew of no one else my age with such a passionate interest in astronomy and the universe.

I often asked my parents about science, but they were unable to answer any of my questions. Their lack of any formal education made it impossible to even comprehend what I was asking. My dad attempted to converse with me in Italian, and I was always impressed with his logical reasoning despite his lack of knowledge. Mom, on the other hand, rarely attempted any discussion. Instead, she would tell me she did not know and that I should ask my teachers in school.

One of the earliest questions I frequently ran by my parents was whether or not the universe had an end. Mom would tell me to go out and play, whereas Dad would repeatedly say that there must be an end, although he could not imagine what the end consisted of. But I would always insist that the universe can have no end, that it must continue on and on. I was so curious that sometimes, I wouldn't be able to fall asleep at night because I was rapt in the struggle to grasp the concept of an infinite universe. I would keep thinking out loud, *Space must be something; it can't be nothing. If one could stick one's hand into space, then how could that space be the end of the universe?"*

Whenever I was tutored by Mr. Kirsch, I would run the same question by him. His answer was that it is likely that the universe is, indeed, without an end. He also told me that he was not a physicist and that I would learn more about the subject later in my education when I was taught about Albert Einstein. That was the first time I had heard the name Albert Einstein.

Another nagging question for my mom and dad related to the topic of the speed by which sound and light travel. One evening during dinner, I asked my parents, "Do sound and light travel in the air at the same speed?"

Mom responded, "Don't talk while you're eating," whereas Dad said, "Let's wait until after dinner to talk about it."

Soon after dinner, my dad asked me why I was so curious about the speed of sound and light. "What difference does it make? Why is that so important to know?" he asked.

"Dad," I said, "I'm just trying to understand what sound and light are made of because I think that light moves faster than sound."

"Why do you think so?" he asked.

"When I see a police car on the street race by at nearly 100 mph, with its siren blasting, it seems like the sounds of the engine and siren are behind the police car. While I'm standing on the sidewalk looking at the police car, the car goes by first, followed by the sounds of the car and siren. The sounds are not keeping up with the car."

"That's not possible, son," my dad said with conviction.

"Dad, I have an idea about an experiment I want to do, but I need your help. Will you help me?"

"Yes, of course. What are we going to do?"

"I'll explain it to you tomorrow after I think about it some more."

The following morning, I walked down the stairs into the basement, where my dad kept all his tools, paint, and other supplies for work. I went to fetch two items. One was a powerful flashlight, and the other was a battery-operated horn that made an incredibly deafening "ahooga" sound when the button was pressed. I found them both and tested them to be certain they worked. The flashlight was nice and bright, and the horn nearly blew my ears out. I quickly concluded that it was not a good idea to test the horn in the confines of a basement.

Dad returned home from work at about 5:00 p.m. As he walked upstairs into the kitchen, I asked him if he would help me with my experiment once we finished dinner, and he agreed. I showed him the flashlight and horn that we would use as part of the experiment, but he had no idea how we would use them.

We walked about three blocks to an abandoned alleyway that was nearly a half-mile in length. At the far end of the road was a large building, the Long Beach Public Bus Terminal, which was empty and abandoned. I explained our experiment to him.

"Dad, I want you to hold the flashlight in one hand and hold the horn in the other hand. Then, I'm going to run to the opposite end of the alleyway. You wait for my signal, I'll say *va bene* (okay, in Italian), and you press the button for the flashlight at exactly the same time that you press the button for the horn. Remember, it is very important that you press the button for the flashlight at **exactly** the same time that you press the button for the horn."

"But what will you do at the other end of the street?" Dad inquired.

"You aim both the flashlight and the horn directly at me, so that I can see the light beam and hear the horn from the other end, far away, okay?"

"Di cosa stai parlando?" *What are you talking about?*

"Don't worry about it now. I promise to explain everything to you when we finish."

I ran all the way down the alleyway to the other end. While running, I realized that the sun had set and it was quite dark—a perfect setting for my experiment. I needed a clear view of the beam of light from the flashlight. I held no doubt that I would hear the ahooga horn, loud and clear.

I looked up the alleyway at my dad, but I couldn't see him. It was too dark out. I yelled out at the top of my lungs, "*Va bene!*" and waited. Then it happened. "Oh my God," I said out loud. "It worked!"

The light beam appeared first. Then, about a second or so later, I heard the loud blast of the horn. The experiment was a success in that the results proved, at least to me, that light travels faster than sound. But I needed to be certain. Suppose Dad had turned on the flashlight one second before sounding the horn? That procedure would clearly have explained the results.

And so, I ran back to him and told him that we needed to repeat the experiment a few more times.

"Ma perché dobbiamo farlo di nuovo?" *But why must we do it again?*

After explaining, I asked him to repeat the experiment three more times, about thirty seconds apart. "Dad, it's too far to keep running back and forth to explain what to do. After I say 'okay' the first time, wait a half-minute or so and do the same thing again. Let's do it three more times."

I ran back to the far end of the road and signaled my dad to turn on both the flashlight and horn. Patiently, I awaited the results of the repeat experiments. *Fantastic,* I thought. In every single case, I saw the flashlight beam about a second before I could hear the sound of the horn.

However, I still needed to do one more essential part of the experiment. I jogged back to my dad and told him that we needed to do this once more, but this time, I would stand only fifteen or twenty feet away. Sure enough, as I expected, the beam of light appeared at exactly the same time as the sound from the horn.

On the way home, I explained the experimental results to Dad. It took him a few minutes to comprehend what I was describing, but then he said, "Capisco—si, capisco." *I understand—yes, I understand.*

I was so thrilled that my dad understood what I had proven. That meant so much to me at the time, and I still think about it today. My father had no formal education whatsoever, not even making it to the first grade, and yet he now understood that light travels faster than sound. Of course, he didn't understand why, but neither did I, for that matter, at the age of ten years.

Chapter 2:
My First Hands-on Experience with Science

B y the fifth grade, I appeared to be in control of my own destiny. My grades had improved, as had my English, both spoken and written. I developed a growing interest in and passion for chemistry and biology. I found these subjects fascinating, and I could not read enough books about chemistry and biology, even though it was years before I would be presented with these subjects in school. I often reflect back and wonder why I had such an interest in these areas. While all my close friends were interested in history, geography, music, art, or English literature, I stood alone, buried in my love of science.

Motivation and perseverance were two traits I possessed early on. My mom often took my brother and me to the local beach, where I learned how to build sandcastles using wet sand near the water's edge. The technique was to grab a pile of very wet sand near the water's edge and allow it to drip down into columns of varying widths. With a foundation established, I could make individual columns and, after some effort, fabricate a castle with many rooms. I labored for hours as my mom kept rubbing sunscreen on my back and arms to prevent sunburn. The sandcastles projected proudly into the sky until the rising tide rushed in and melted down what I had spent hours building up. *No problem*, I thought, *I'll just build another one tomorrow.*

I built my largest sandcastle ever on a July 4 weekend. I started early, at about 8:00 a.m., but before I could finish construction, the city workers told me I had to vacate the area because they were about to set up the fireworks display. I was disappointed at first, but soon I became enthralled by the multitude of fireworks.

We went home for dinner and returned to the beach after dark to watch the fireworks. We weren't allowed near the launching site, but I positioned myself close enough to watch the action quite clearly. The noise, fire, and lights were something to see. I have never forgotten that fireworks display. Indeed, I became eager to set up such a display in my own backyard.

The Long Beach Public Library was only a few blocks from home, and I spent some time there, reading about fireworks. Although I experienced great difficulty in understanding most of what I was reading, I realized that a chemistry set might help me achieve my goal. In considering my plan of attack, I knew that I had to convince my mom and dad to buy me a chemistry set—a big one.

This was not going to be easy because my mom was always careful about what I was and wasn't allowed to do at home. Although not a terribly mischievous child, I was no angel either, and Mom was the disciplinarian. Whenever I got into trouble, she would run after me, but I was too fast for her to catch me. She finally learned how to get me—she'd remove her heavy wooden slipper and throw the perfect curve, sending it sailing through the air where it would go around the corner into the room I had entered and clock me in the back of the head.

In 1951, at ten years old, I finally got the courage to ask my mom and dad to buy me a chemistry set. They wanted to know why I wanted a chemistry set at such a young age—too young, they guessed, to be able to read and understand what I was doing.

I answered, "So I can learn some chemistry and better understand the makeup of solids, liquids, and gases."

My parents were dumbfounded by my response.

Mom jumped in first, "What are you talking about? No, you cannot have a chemistry set! You are way too young for such things."

Dad cut in with, "Okay, let us think about it for a while."

But Mom interrupted, shouting, "I said no! There will be no chemistry set in this house, and that's final!"

Later that afternoon, I overheard my dad telling Mom, in Italian, that I should have a chemistry set and anything else I wanted that would better my education.

"Don't you see that our son wants to do things that we never even heard of before?" he said. "How can you say no to that? You should have seen when Louie showed me that light moves faster than sound. That was truly amazing. I would never have guessed it."

Mom said abruptly that a chemistry set would be too danger-ous for a ten-year-old, and I might hurt myself or someone else. Later, they both approached me and asked me exactly what I planned to do with the chemicals. I told them I was going to read the booklet of instructions and mix certain chemicals according to the directions and then observe the results. "These are called experiments, and they are safe for children," I added.

A few moments later, Mom and Dad looked at each other and told me they would buy me a chemistry set provided I followed the directions "exactly" and "very carefully."

I knew exactly which one I wanted. Having already done my research, I directed my mom to the exact place in the aisle at the hobby store. The tag read, "Gilbert Chemistry Set."

After some hesitation, Mom said, "My God, this is a lot of money. If you really want this, it will be your birthday present, and you won't get anything else for your birthday. Do you un-derstand that?"

"Yes, Mom. I understand."

When I first opened my chemistry set, I looked at all the chemicals and mixing and measuring supplies that were included. Then I took out the instruction booklet and read it from cover to cover. I became fascinated with the way different chemicals reacted under different experimental conditions.

Of course, I hadn't *exactly* told them the whole truth. My true motivation and intentions were to make firecrackers and rocket fuel. And, after performing each of the experiments outlined in the booklet, I set out to do just that.

Alfred Nobel

During my course of reading library books about explosives, I frequently ran across the name Alfred Nobel.

Alfred Bernhard Nobel was born on October 21, 1833, in Stockholm, Sweden. He was one of eight children, and the fourth son of Immanuel and Caroline Nobel. In the early- to mid-1800s, life was nearly intolerable for Swedes who were poor, and that included the Nobel family.

As Alfred grew, he became inquisitive, full of intellectual curiosity, and constantly asked questions. By the age of ten, he had developed a keen interest in chemistry and explosives. This interest grew out of his father's profession as a manufacturer of explosive mines for warfare. Nobel (similar to yours truly) was determined to read as much as he could on his own about chemistry, and in a relatively short period, Alfred learned that gunpowder was a mixture of sulfur, charcoal powder, and saltpeter (another name for potassium nitrate or KNO_3).

Alfred had no formal education in elementary or high school. He had excellent tutors, especially in chemistry, particularly Professor Yuli Trapp, who was the first to introduce Alfred to a new explosive, nitroglycerin. Nitroglycerin was powerful but highly unstable. Exposing nitroglycerin to heat, sunlight, or simple agitation could result in spontaneous detonation with grave consequences. At the time, the only dependable explosive for use in mines was "black powder," a form of gunpowder.

Nobel reasoned that nitroglycerin would be the ideal explosive for the Nobel family business, which was heavy construction and demolition for mining and building transportation networks, such as roads and tunnels. However, Ascanio Sobrero, the original inventor of nitroglycerin, opposed the use of the unpredictable and unstable substance as an explosive for use in mines because he considered it too dangerous to be of any practical use. Nevertheless, Nobel wanted to find a way to control and use nitroglycerin not only for the family business but also as a commercial explosive.

By 1862, Alfred had begun experimenting with nitroglycerin in a small laboratory on his father's estate in Stockholm. He found that when nitroglycerin was carefully incorporated into an absorbent, inert substance like *kieselguhr* (diatomaceous earth), it became more stable. The kieselguhr allowed the liquid nitroglycerin to be absorbed to dryness, and the resulting mixture was safer to handle, transport, and use than nitroglycerin alone. Satisfied with this discovery, he experimented further to come up with a safe way to control detonation.

In 1864, Nobel invented an improved detonator called a blasting cap, which inaugurated the modern use of high explosives. It was one of the defining moments that led to the fortune he would go on to acquire as a manufacturer of powerful explosives. Some asserted he was in too much of a hurry to exploit his invention, which was very dangerous and could result in grave consequences. He was about to discover that the cost of being a pioneer could be tragically high.

Saturday, September 3, 1864, promised to be a beautiful early autumn day. In a small backyard laboratory, which was actually a shed located a few meters from the main house, Emil Nobel,

Alfred's younger brother, was busy purifying large quantities of nitroglycerin for an order from the local railway company. After several months of work, a large stock of nitroglycerin, about 250 pounds, had been prepared and stored in the laboratory shed. During that time, the neighbors felt that they were living on top of a volcano, and they complained to the landlord on many occasions.

The yard outside the main building was deserted when catastrophe struck. The laboratory in the shed exploded with a thunderous roar. According to the report in the newspaper, the force was so violent *"that the buildings shook on their foundations and windows in places around Kungsholm shattered."*

The article in the newspaper continues: *"We would learn later that the source of the blast was a building on the Heleneborg estate at Langholm Bay, where the engineer Nobel had constructed a nitroglycerin factory. In the capital people heard the violent sound of the explosion and saw a huge, yellow flame rise straight up in the air … A much more terrible sight awaited one at the site of the accident. There was nothing left of the factory, a wooden building adjacent to the Heleneborg estate, except a few charred fragments thrown here and there. In the houses nearby, and even those on the other side of the bay, not only had the glass panes been smashed but also windowsills and molding."*

Nobel was devastated by the nitroglycerin explosion. Anxious to prevent additional accidents, Nobel developed research centers to focus specifically on improving the stability of the explosives he was developing. He experimented and found that his mixture could be maintained safely when wrapped in warm, soft wax and fitted with a fuse, and he patented this invention in 1867 as "dynamite," named from the Greek *dynamis* or "power."

Despite this incredibly monumental invention, the explosion at Heleneborg would reverberate in the minds of Stockholm's citizens for decades. Indeed, the people often referred to local events as occurring before or after *"the Nobel bang."*

I spent several months reading up on how Nobel had prepared different mixtures of gunpowder by varying the ratios of three compounds: sulfur, charcoal powder, and potassium nitrate. I also discovered these were the same ingredients required to make firecrackers and rocket fuel.

Okay, I thought, *I'm ready to go!* However, I ran into one critical obstacle. The chemistry set came with a very limited quantity of sulfur, and the two other ingredients I needed were not included at all. Now what was I going to do?

At this time, I first heard about nitroglycerin as an explosive. Dynamite was quite familiar to me, but I did not realize that the active explosive in dynamite was nitroglycerin. What confused me was that one of our close neighbors, Samuel Abrahams, had been taking nitroglycerin tablets to treat his chest pains or angina pectoris. And so, I had come to believe that nitroglycerin was a drug, not an explosive.

In reading up on nitroglycerin, I again came across the name Alfred Nobel. Not only did I realize that nitroglycerin was both an explosive and a medication to treat heart ailments, but I also was introduced to the Nobel Prize and that it was awarded to distinguished people in the name of Alfred Nobel.

As I read further, I thought perhaps nitroglycerin might be easier to prepare or purchase than the ingredients to make gunpowder. But I learned that nitroglycerin was a terribly dangerous and highly explosive chemical and determined that it probably would not be ideal for making a firecracker or rocket fuel. Besides, one could not purchase nitroglycerin alone because it tended to explode spontaneously. Clearly, my mom would not approve such a purchase.

I concluded that gunpowder was the only route to make my fireworks and rocket fuel.

Now, where to get it? In my readings, I noted that such chemicals were carried by, and available from, local pharmacies. Back in those days, most drugs did not come ready-made or formulated in dosages that could be transferred to a bottle for sale to customers. Instead, pharmacists had to "compound" most prescriptions as ordered by the doctor, so they had lots of chemicals on hand.

I asked my mom to take me to the drug store the next time she needed to make a purchase there. When she asked me why, I told her that I was interested in chemicals, and I wanted to see the chemicals that a pharmacy carries.

At the shop, I walked around and looked at the shelves to see what I could find. One of the pharmacists asked me if I was looking for anything special. I told him that I was interested in chemicals and medicines and what the bottles or containers looked like. The pharmacist took me behind the counter and showed me the chemicals he used to fill prescriptions. And there they were: large containers of sulfur, charcoal powder, and potassium nitrate. I couldn't believe my eyes when I saw those large containers!

On the walk home, I began thinking about how I would obtain those three chemicals from the pharmacy. Suddenly, it came to me. One of my close friends, Steve, had an older brother, Alan, who had a summer job at our local pharmacy. I asked Steve to introduce me to his older brother, and I seized that opportunity to ask him if he was allowed to buy chemicals from the pharmacy.

"I don't see why not," Alan said. I told him that I was engaged in a chemistry project, and I needed some sulfur, charcoal powder, and potassium nitrate. Alan asked me for some money and went off to see what he could do. When Alan returned, he told me that the pharmacist sold him the sulfur and charcoal powder but would not sell him any potassium nitrate. The pharmacist had suspected that Alan intended to use potassium nitrate to make rocket fuel and wouldn't sell him any.

I kept thinking about how I was going to get ahold of potassium nitrate, which was vital to the completion of my project. Then, one morning, Alan appeared with a container of potassium nitrate and told me I owed him five bucks. After thanking him, I asked him how he was able to buy it. He said he'd asked one of his friends to buy it for him. Apparently, the pharmacist did not make the connection to Alan's previous purchase.

Once armed with the necessary ingredients, I used a simple mixture of sulfur, charcoal powder, and potassium nitrate (similar to a mixture Nobel had used), and I succeeded in making a powder mixture that burned rapidly when ignited. I figured that the mixture would be an ideal rocket fuel. Through my experiments, I had found that inserting a fuse and lighting the opposite end made the burning more reproducible and controllable. These fuses were strings composed of fine paper (readily available in hobby shops) that had been twisted in gunpowder. I used this fuse as a type of detonator to ignite my gunpowder mixture, similar to a fuse detonator Alfred Nobel had used when he invented dynamite.

My dad also got into the act, and I was pleased about that. He built a small, lightweight rocket using balsa wood. I used Dad's roll of pliable aluminum sheet metal to make a small, elongated chamber to contain the rocket fuel mixture. In addition, my dad constructed a suitable launching platform, with a guide firmly mounted to it, that would serve to guide the rocket upward in what we hoped would be a straight trajectory.

The day of the launch finally came. I was excited and anxious all morning, waiting for Dad to return home for his lunch break. I hoped that our home-built rocket would travel at least several stories up into the air. Moreover, I was already thinking about how I could modify the gunpowder mixture to make it even more powerful. My dad pulled up and walked up the driveway straight to the backyard, where he had positioned the launching platform.

"Va bene, facciamolo," he said. *Okay, let's do it.*

I inserted the fuse into the small hole at the bottom of the fuel chamber and then lit the free end, which was dangling down about three inches below the platform. The fuse ignited perfectly, and four or five seconds later, when the flame reached the mixture in the chamber, the rocket took off at lightning speed.

Unfortunately, the predicted trajectory was a bit off, and the rocket quickly veered left and went straight through my next-door neighbor's side window.

My dad did a great job replacing our neighbor's window the next morning. Because my dad had been present during the launch, our neighbor was not upset.

"Accidents happen," Dad said. "We'll do a much better job next time."

My mother, on the other hand, argued that the horrible incident would never have happened had I not messed around with a chemistry set.

Then she asked the key question: "Louie, show me right now the page in the chemistry booklet that explains how to make what you just made!"

"Well," I said, "there's not exactly any *one page* that gives those directions. I just got that idea from reading many experiments in other chemistry books and then figuring out how to make rocket fuel."

Mom gave me a penetrating stare that could have drilled a hole in the wall.

Mom reminded Dad that I was too young to play with explosive chemicals and that I would seriously hurt myself. But she never yelled at him. Mom and Dad never raised their voices at each other in my presence.

A two-month cease-fire followed, which included a series of discussions with Mom. She tried to explain that "shooting up rocket ships" could actually kill somebody.

"Louie," she once said to me, "suppose the rocket ship comes down near the sidewalk or street and hits somebody on the head? Then what?"

But I was not done with my gunpowder mixtures, not by a long shot. Instead of rocket fuel, I attempted to make a firecracker using basically the same explosive mixture, but this time the mixture was contained within a paper straw that I sealed at one end and fitted a fuse into the opposite end.

To avoid startling my neighbors, especially the one next door, I chose to ignite the fuse in an open lot a few blocks from home. I did this on a weekend morning at about 6:00 a.m.

Success! It sounded just like a real firecracker, although not as loud. I was less than impressed with the meager crackling sound and absence of any destructive force. I was hoping for a much louder pop, accompanied by dirt flying into the air. I proceeded to read more chemistry books that I checked out of our local library, and I experimented with various gunpowder mixtures that I prepared from scratch.

These upgraded gunpowder formulations required that I purchase new chemicals. My shopping list expanded to include ammonium nitrate and coarsely powdered magnesium ribbon. Ammonium nitrate is a component of fertilizer but is also a powerful explosive under certain conditions, including high heat. Magnesium ribbon, when pulverized to a coarse powder, will ignite under high temperatures and burn extremely rapidly, thereby creating a great deal of pressure or force.

Once again, I asked Alan to purchase these chemicals from the neighborhood pharmacy. He was successful, and I was ready to make and test my new formula. But this time, I did not use a flimsy paper straw.

My dad had a fairly extensive assortment of copper tubing that he used on the job. I chose one that was more flexible (thinner walls). I placed the mixture into the copper tubing, capped it with a twist cap on one end, and tapered the other end to be fitted with a fuse. Then, I waited until my parents left home and elected to ignite my invention in the basement within a tightly locked dresser drawer that my mom used to store our extra heavy winter underwear and socks. I figured this would muffle the sound. I also imagined I'd get to witness whether or not the exploding firecracker had enough force to push open the dresser drawers.

Upon detonation, I realized I had made a mistake. A very big mistake. Turned out, my modified firecracker was more like a small bomb. It totaled the dresser from top to bottom and scattered the underwear and socks throughout the entire basement. Luckily, the flying splinters barely missed me, as I was standing only about ten feet away. But I did feel the impact of the flying underwear.

I needed to act fast to clean up the basement. I threw away the damaged clothes that had black and yellow stains from the blast and folded and put away the ones I could salvage in another dresser nearby. I then put the scraps of the destroyed dresser in the trash outside. The next day, I explained to my dad what I had done, and all he asked was that I be careful and not blow up the house ... and that I not tell my mom about this incident. As far as I know, Mom never found out what I had accomplished while she was away those few hours.

Although I was fairly impressed with my new explosive mixture, I could not tell how loud this beefed-up firecracker was because the sound was muffled. The force of the explosion was evident, but that may have been because the firecracker was sealed within the dresser. I had to set off the next firecracker outdoors.

And so, I modified the first mixture by adding a bit more ammonium nitrate, and I carefully placed the mixture into a larger piece of copper pipe that I found in my dad's scrap pile of assorted used pipe. This time, the copper pipe had thicker walls.

Again, after sealing one end and placing a fuse into the opposite end, I decided to detonate my invention in the backyard. But I needed to find a spot that could withstand the potential explosive nature of my new invention. I decided on the grilling portion of a brick fireplace that my dad had just built as a family barbecue Dad had put in about a month's work on weekends to construct the fireplace in the late spring so that it would be ready for use by summer.

The bar-b-que was constructed of layers of solid red firebrick and reinforced with rebar. I was convinced that the structure was more than solid enough to withstand the impact of my modified firecracker.

How wrong I was! Upon detonation, the entire back wall of the brick fireplace detached, projected backward, and quickly found its way into my neighbor's yard, just missing their garage but demolishing their lawnmower shed. How was I going to explain this to Mom and Dad, especially my dad, since I'd blown apart all his hard work?

Once again, my dad was impressed with my explosive skills, whereas my mom was concerned about my destructive ones. She took to her slipper trick and chased me out of the house. As I was running for my life, she screamed, "And don't you come back home until you behave!"

I managed to make peace with my dad. Mom, on the other hand, was getting fed up with me, so I decided to take a hiatus from bomb designing for about a year.

One of my less destructive (yet equally creative) hobbies as a child was model railroading. It all started one morning in 1953, at the age of twelve, when I went with my dad to a local hardware store. I vividly recall the name of the hardware store: Greenberg's Hardware. Being a carpenter, my dad frequently purchased materials there. One day in early December as Christmas was approaching, I accompanied him. I walked into the store and was immediately attracted to a large model railroad display, complete with running trains and lighted buildings. I remained fixed to the display while my dad did his shopping.

Later that evening, at the dinner table, my dad asked me if I liked the trains at the hardware store. I told him I did and asked him if it was okay if I occasionally walked to Greenberg's by myself to look at the trains. Mom approved, as long as I was extra careful crossing the streets. For obvious reasons, she preferred model trains over my chemistry set.

After I made a series of visits to the hardware store, the owner told my dad that I had spent many hours examining the train layout to see how it was all put together, including the electric wiring. Dad surprised me by asking if I would like to have a small train set at home. He said that I could set it up in our basement after he cleared away some old furniture. We went to the store, and I picked out a Lionel train set. On returning home, my dad spent a few hours building a tabletop for my trains. The rest was up to me. I read the instruction manual, and after a few hours, turned on the power transformer. I locomotive started moving the freight train around the oval layout. I ran upstairs to get my mom to come down and see what I had done. She was impressed. When Dad came home, he, too, was impressed, mainly because I'd connected all the wires properly.

Over the next few weeks, I went to local hobby stores to learn how to construct hills and tunnels from paper mâché. I used my dad's paints to give the fixtures some color, and used sand, soil, and dried grass from outdoors to add more realism to the layout. Dad asked me if I wanted a larger layout. Without hesitation, I agreed, and he built another tabletop of equal size and attached it to the initial table.

Although I'd become involved with trains, I did not forget my passion about understanding the chemistry of fireworks and rocket fuel. Something about how chemicals reacted with each other captured my imagination at such a young age. How does a chemical reaction cause fire or an explosion? Mom always used a mixture of baking powder and vinegar to scrub the sink. When she combined the two, the mixture would fizz and bubble. I was always interested in the chemistry of the reaction. Why did the mixture fizz and bubble?

Chemistry, however, was not the only science in which I had a keen interest. One morning, I found a squirrel that had just been attacked and killed by a cat. It appeared the cat had broken the squirrel's neck. I seized the opportunity to dissect the animal's abdomen and have a look inside. The arrangement of the internal organs looked just like that in humans, so I ran to my room to fetch my human anatomy textbook, which my neighbor had given me. What impressed me so much was that the arrangement (gross anatomy) of the digestive and circulatory systems in the squirrel was so similar to that of humans. Much to my mom's dismay, I spent the next few months searching for more dead animals to dissect.

It seemed that anything and everything in science appealed to me. This was most definitely not the case with any of my schoolmates or neighbors, who showed absolutely no interest in anything I had to say about science. Indeed, they often asked me, "Why are you so gung-ho over that stuff?"

During the waiting period since my brick fireplace explosion, I engaged myself in more in-depth reading pertaining to what ingredients make up a good, homemade bomb. In those days, there were no organized terrorists with plastic explosives, hydroperoxides, or anything close to that. I simply used the standard gunpowder ingredients, legally obtainable at any local pharmacy, to which I added a few new chemicals. If I were to make a more explosive mixture, finding the appropriate proportions of all ingredients was the key. *After all,* I thought, *this is what Alfred Nobel did in his laboratory in Stockholm when he experimented with gunpowder.*

After my year-long hiatus from experimenting with explosives, I thought I would have one more attempt at making a bomb that would finally satisfy my curiosity. I wanted to see if I could make one with more destructive capacity, such as causing a small crater in the ground.

I carefully incorporated finely ground magnesium powder, which I already had, and potassium permanganate, which I had to get my friends to buy for me. I'd learned that potassium permanganate (sold as a topical antiseptic) reacts slowly with glycerin (used by pharmacists to give a sweet taste to otherwise bitter solutions for oral consumption) to form a powerful oxidizing substance that ignites spontaneously after a few minutes.

Ah ha, I thought. *This should make a good delayed fuse and give me ample time to make my escape before detonation.* After experimenting with tiny amounts of my mixture in an open crucible, I was ready to pack several tablespoons of my mix into a four-inch section of lead pipe (about a half-inch in diameter) that was sealed with a cap on one end. The opposite end was fitted with a cap through which I had drilled a one-eighth-inch hole to insert my homemade delayed fuse.

I only had one remaining consideration: where to detonate this thing?

For sure, I was not going to try this anywhere near home or my neighbors. The local beach came to mind. It had a three-mile stretch of boardwalk, held up by a large array of concrete pillars, each about two feet square and eight feet tall. It was the same stretch of boardwalk where my father had supervised the rebuild project in the 1930s.

I rode my bike to the boardwalk and walked on the sand to examine the pillars underneath. I noticed that some pillars had holes about two inches in diameter that protruded about one foot into the pillar before ending at the surface of the steel substructure. Why some pillars had these holes was not obvious to me, but I figured that such a hole would be a convenient spot to plant my pipe bomb.

And so, the next morning, bright and early at sunrise, I took my experiment with me on my bike and inserted the pipe into the hole of one of the pillars. The long fuse was a segment of narrow rope that had been soaked overnight in potassium permanganate solution. I was then ready to submerge the free end of the rope into a vial of liquid glycerin. But before that, I climbed up to the boardwalk to be certain no one was walking close by or even in sight for at least two blocks. Also, I made sure that my bike was near and upright, ready for me to mount and take off promptly after ignition.

The time had finally come. A full year had gone by without my setting off an explosive, not even a firecracker. What was I to expect from my homemade invention? Well, there was only one way to find out. I made the contact between the potassium permanganate and glycerin, ran full speed to my bike, mounted it, and rode off as fast as my legs would take me on the street that parallels the boardwalk and beach. After four long blocks away, I turned left onto Long Beach Road and was about to head home. But first, I stopped for a moment to listen for an explosion, which had not yet occurred. I thought that perhaps my delayed fuse did not work properly ...

Suddenly, a deep explosive roar ripped through the air with the sound of a collapsing building. *Oh my God*, I thought. *I'm nearly a mile from the detonation site, and I can hear and feel the sound as if I were fifty feet away!*

Now I was scared. *What have I done? Was anybody hurt?* Had anybody walked onto the boardwalk after I'd fled the scene? Was there still a boardwalk above that pillar? The one thing I knew for sure was that I had to get home, quickly put my bike away in the basement, enter the rear door of my house, and pretend I'd been studying in my bedroom.

I made it home quickly and, after a few hours, I began to relax a bit. Then my mom walked into my bedroom.

"Louie," she said, "I suppose you had nothing to do with that enormous blast that occurred at the beach about five hours ago?"

Startled, I looked up at her with the most innocent face I could muster and said, "No, Mom. What blast? I didn't hear anything."

She looked at me, gave me her typical Mona Lisa smile, and said, "Good."

But I knew from her expression that she did not believe me one bit. I suspected that she didn't have enough evidence to convict me, at least not yet. The rest of the day was nerve-racking, as I feared the news of a terrible explosion under the boardwalk, with people injured as a result. But the entire day and evening went by without any word of the explosion. After watching TV for an hour or so, I went to bed, relieved that no one had been hurt. In addition, it was truly comforting to escape being slammed on the back of the head with a curveball slipper.

I was anxious to return to the beach to see the results of my experiment, but I decided to wait a few weeks in case the local police were at the site conducting an investigation. About six weeks later, I rode my bike to the beach and stopped on the sidewalk about a hundred feet away from the pillar of detonation.

I couldn't believe my eyes. The pillar containing my pipe bomb was totally cleared of any visible concrete; only bare steel remained. I walked up to the pillar and noticed that the concrete debris had been cleared away. So, someone obviously had noticed the destruction and cleaned up the mess. What was even more frightening was the appearance of the pillar to the left of the pillar containing the bomb. This adjacent pillar was about ten feet away and had a big chunk of concrete missing. Embedded in the concrete remaining on that adjacent pillar was the metal cap from the lead pipe I used for the bomb. Apparently, upon explosion, the cap stripped the threads on the main pipe, rocketed out of the hole in a straight line to the adjacent pillar, knocked out a big section of concrete, and embedded itself into the pillar. Suddenly, I realized the magnitude of what I had built at just fourteen years of age. I left quietly, rode home, and never again entertained the notion of playing around with explosives.

Chapter 3:

Drag Racing and Linus Pauling

After completing my second year in high school and approaching the end of summer vacation, my close friend Russ Wayne invited me over for lunch at his home, located about five blocks away from mine. His home was large, beautiful, and situated in the nicest part of Long Beach. But what I remember most about their home was the large garage, which housed a car that Russ's older brother, Jim, used for drag racing at the quarter-mile drag strip in Westhampton, Long Island. Jim was an excellent mechanic who spent a lot of time modifying and tuning up his 1956 Ford Fairlane. In those days, the car to beat at the drag strip was the Chevrolet Impala packed with a powerful V8 engine, but Jim knew just how to modify and tune up his Ford to beat any Chevy.

The sounds of fast cars had been catching my attention more and more since I'd given up making bombs. The roar of the engines from souped-up coupes made my head turn every time they raced by. Something was satisfying about the explosive sounds made by internal combustion engines, which all cars had at the time. Particularly intriguing to me was the deep, soothing purring sound of a V8 engine, especially in a car that had been modified by replacing standard mufflers, allowing more sound to pass through.

I was determined to learn about the internal combustion engine and how it could be modified to make it develop more horsepower. To my way of thinking, although this was mechanics, it was still science because the more one experimented, the more one understood the process. I had always found that experimentation was the best way to learn.

Jim let me watch him work on his engine and tune it up nearly every weekend. He saw that I was interested in what he was doing, so he asked me to help him remove the carburetor and intake manifold, both of which sit on top of the engine. I observed as Jim tuned the valves and carefully replaced the gaskets.

Then, he trusted me to replace the valve covers and install a new intake manifold, which could accommodate two individual two-barrel carburetors, instead of the single one that was present in the standard vehicle. Jim installed the carburetors himself but showed me how to tune them up to work together in a synchronous manner. I quickly learned that one of the best ways to know whether the engine was properly tuned was the smooth purring sound that only a well-tuned engine can make. Russ later told me that Jim was impressed with my skills.

I worked with Jim on several occasions after that, and he and his racing buddies invited Russ and me to the Westhampton Raceway for drag racing. It housed a typical quarter-mile drag strip with an official starter (flagman) and electronic sensor devices at the finish line to determine both speed (mph) and elapsed time (seconds).

I was so excited to be present and watch the various classes of cars race down the strip. There were standard (not significantly modified) cars and modified cars. Some vehicles were classified as dragsters, which are so drastically modified that they are not considered to be cars. The dragsters were always the fastest vehicles on the track. The smell of engines running, gasoline fumes, nitro-gasoline mixtures, and the rubber that burned under the tires as the cars and dragsters accelerated from the starting line was a thrill that I could not get out of my system for many years to come.

Meeting Linus Pauling

Upon starting the eleventh grade that fall, I quickly recognized that, although we had a course in chemistry, no laboratory component was associated with the lectures. That was most disappointing to me. Lab work was what I was most looking forward to. I approached my general science/chemistry teacher and asked him why physics had a lab, but chemistry did not. I explained that we would probably learn more from laboratory work than from lectures only. My teacher agreed and apologized that the school had no chem lab.

A few weeks later, my teacher approached me again and asked if I would be interested in helping him set up a chemistry laboratory, which would be taught in the following year. Even though I would not be able to take the chem lab in my senior year due to other academic obligations, I knew what an incredible learning experience it would be to help set it up, and I enthusiastically accepted.

My teacher told me that a famous chemist would be coming to our high school for a few days to help us set up the chem lab and also demonstrate exciting experiments in science and chemistry, and that I would be working with him. He revealed that our guest would be Professor Linus Pauling.

Upon hearing that, my mouth dropped open. "Didn't Professor Pauling win the Nobel Prize a couple of years ago?" I asked.

Pauling had been awarded the Nobel Prize in Chemistry in 1954, two years prior. *Incredible*, I thought. *I'm going to spend some time with a Nobel Prize-winning chemist.*

The day my teacher introduced Professor Pauling to our chemistry class, I was struck with his appearance as he entered the room. In his fifties at the time, he stood at least six feet tall and had bushy, gray-white hair with bulging eyes. Our teacher explained that Professor Pauling was a famous chemist who had been awarded the Nobel Prize for his basic research in chemistry, more specifically, the chemical bond.

Dr. Pauling began by telling us about himself and how his passion for chemistry began when he was a young child. It reminded me of my own early interest in chemistry. He told the class that he had been most interested in the composition of matter. As he said that, I recounted in my own mind my childhood interest in the composition of explosives.

Professor Pauling became quite excited as he explained that molecules consist of atoms, which, in turn, consist of protons, neutrons, and electrons. He continued by telling us that the combination of, or reaction between, different atoms creates different molecules and that understanding the properties of atoms allows one to understand the composition of matter.

He spoke with a smile in a soft-spoken voice that carried across the classroom. His manner of speaking commanded the attention of everyone listening. His presentation was lucid and easy to follow.

Professor Pauling introduced us to the periodic table of chemical elements. To assist him, our teacher mounted a large cardboard illustration of the periodic table onto a tripod in front of the classroom. He explained that the periodic table consists of horizontal rows and vertical columns of the known ninety-eight elements. Then he asked the class a question: "What is the purpose or significance of this tabular illustration of the chemical elements? How does this arrangement of elements help you to understand the properties and reactivity of the elements in nature?"

The room remained silent for several seconds. No one raised a hand to be called on. I had always been fascinated with the periodic table and had studied it time and time again outside the classroom. My teacher and I had previously engaged in several discussions about the chemical properties of the elements, and he knew that I had a keen understanding of the periodic table.

I was going to raise my hand but was suddenly overcome by shyness and trepidation, which is unlike me. I wasn't afraid of speaking in front of my classmates; it had never been a problem for me in the past. Perhaps my feelings could be attributed to the presence of an esteemed Nobel Prize winner. The thought of speaking in front of him was nerve-racking.

The classroom was still quiet when my teacher called upon me. "Mr. Ignarro, would you like to *volunteer* to answer Professor Pauling's question?"

I realized at this point that the word "volunteer" had an entirely new meaning.

Despite being nervous, I agreed to answer.

Dr. Pauling looked over at me and said, "Good. Very well, Mr. Ignarro, would you tell us a little about the periodic table of elements? For example, what kind of useful information about the elements can be derived from the table?" He pointed at the cardboard illustration of the periodic table as he spoke.

"Okay, Professor Pauling, I'll try my best."

I was still sitting at my desk when I started to give my answer. The teacher quickly interrupted me, "Mr. Ignarro, would you kindly join us at the front of the class to provide your explanation?"

Now, I was really nervous. I left my seat and came to the front of the room, where I began to speak. By this time, I was so shaken up that I regretted that our teacher had ever called on me. But there I was, standing up in front of the class next to Dr. Pauling, with all eyes in the room on me.

With an audible sigh, I proceeded to explain to the class, and Professor Pauling, that, "The periodic table is a method of organizing the chemical elements to make it easier to see the relationships among the different elements." I continued, "It's like a chart consisting of rows and columns of the elements. The columns contain elements with similar chemical properties because all elements under the same column have the same number of reactive electrons. The rows of elements tell us something different. The elements across a given row have very different chemical properties because these elements have a different number of reactive electrons."

I looked over at our teacher, who was standing in the side aisle of the classroom with a distinct smile on his face. That was a signal that I was doing okay.

I was about to continue by expanding my answer, but I decided to pause because it appeared that Dr. Pauling wanted to say something.

"Very good, Mr. Ignarro. That was an excellent answer. But I have just one more question for you, and I don't expect you to know the answer to this one."

Great, I thought. *Just as I started to calm down ...* My nerves picked up once again.

"Who first conceived of or invented the periodic table of the elements?" Professor Pauling asked.

My heart rate jumped up because I knew the answer. "Professor Mendeleev, from Russia," I answered.

"Yes. Yes. Correct!" Dr. Pauling said.

The entire classroom erupted with whistles and applause. But I also heard snickering from some of my classmates, perhaps because they suspected I was showing off. However, I was concerned only with not making a fool of myself in front of a Nobel Laureate. Later that afternoon, our teacher confided in me that even he had not recalled the name of Mendeleev.

Dr. Pauling went on to demonstrate a few exciting chemistry experiments and then showed us what we needed to set up a bona fide chemistry lab for high school students. His demonstrations were illuminating and mind-capturing. For example, I was intrigued when he mixed together two clear, colorless solutions, and the end result was a red-colored solution. Then he added more of one solution to the other, and it turned blue. This was a demonstration of the famous litmus test in acid/base chemistry.

Another experiment he demonstrated for us showed that one could mix together two clear, colorless solutions and wind up with a white solid material (precipitate). For those of you who are dying to know what the solutions were, one was table salt (sodium chloride) dissolved in water, and the other was a solution of silver nitrate. Mixing the two solutions results in a chemical reaction forming an insoluble compound, silver chloride, and a clear solution of colorless sodium nitrate. The silver atom from silver nitrate reacts with the chloride atom from salt (NaCl) to form silver chloride, which is insoluble in water.

I also vividly recall his discussion and demonstration of how matter can exist in three different phases, depending on the temperature. For example, when water is cooled sufficiently, the water transforms from the liquid phase to the solid phase—ice. When the ice is heated to a high temperature, the ice will transform first back to the liquid phase (water) and then to the gas phase (steam).

That's three different phases. He demonstrated that. Then he asked the question, "How many phases can carbon dioxide gas (CO_2) have?"

Everyone said three phases, but I knew that was incorrect. I said only two phases. Professor Pauling said, "Very good, Mr. Ignarro, but please explain your answer."

And so, I responded, "If you heat up dry ice, which is the solid phase of carbon dioxide, you immediately wind up with carbon dioxide gas, which takes on a whitish color. Carbon dioxide transforms from a solid to a gas, and there is no liquid phase."

"Very good indeed," Dr. Pauling said, "but let's see if you are correct." He proceeded to heat a solid piece of dry ice, and no liquid ever formed; it went directly from solid to gas. He then confirmed, "Yes, you were correct. There's nothing like experimentation to prove a point."

As you can imagine, that made my day. But I did not tell anyone how I'd come to know the answer. It wasn't from a chemistry book. When I was two years younger, I'd had a job selling ice cream from a Good Humor ice cream bike. It was a three-wheeler that had a closed container built into the front end and filled with dry ice to keep the ice cream frozen throughout the day. As the day passed, the dry ice melted, but there was never a drop of liquid anywhere; only the white-colored carbon dioxide gas that escaped into the air.

My experience with Professor Linus Pauling turned out to be the single most important influence in my pursuit of a chemical approach to basic research. This unique, once-in-a-lifetime opportunity instilled in me a passionate desire to study chemistry in college, which was less than two years away.

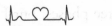

Shortly after my high school experience with Dr. Pauling, and during our junior year physics course and laboratory, I learned that Albert Einstein also had been awarded the Nobel Prize but for his work in physics. Our physics teacher was a big fan of Einstein and devoted several lectures and laboratory exercises to explaining why he was so famous. I also recall him telling us that we could not discuss Einstein's work in great detail because we did not have the mathematical background to do so. Instead, he attempted to explain some of Einstein's work without the math, and he did an excellent job.

$E = mc^2$ is, perhaps, the most famous equation ever conceived. The most exhilarating part of our entire physics course was the two or three days our teacher devoted to the significance of this equation. I was about four years of age when the US dropped an atomic bomb on Hiroshima, Japan, during World War II, and I recall seeing photos and TV videos of the massive destruction it caused. But it was not until now, at sixteen years of age, that I came to realize that the explosive nature of the atomic bomb was attributed to Einstein's famous equation: $E = mc^2$. Simply put, this equation reveals that when mass (m) is changed, the change in energy (E) that results is equivalent to m (mass) multiplied by c^2, as the equation clearly dictates. Since c (the speed of light) is about 670,000,000 miles per hour, it follows that c^2 is $(670,000,000)^2$ or 449,000,000,000,000,000. This means, essentially, that if mass (m) changes by 1 unit, then E changes by 449,00,000,000,000,000 units. Wow! Hence the incredibly destructive nature of the atomic bomb.

What was most attractive to me about $E = mc^2$ was not its destructive potential but rather that experimentation was required to validate Einstein's theory. One simple, albeit destructive, experiment was all that was required to change knowledge from the level of theory to one of incontrovertible scientific fact. I, myself, had found this for all of the experiments I had performed since I was a child.

During our studies of Einstein and the atomic bomb, the subject of radioactivity came up because radioactive uranium isotopes were used in making such bombs. Thus, I learned in class about Madame Marie Curie, who discovered the mechanism of radioactivity and certain new radioactive elements. Not only was she one of the first scientists ever to be awarded the Nobel Prize, but she was also the first woman.

The nature of the accomplishments of Pauling, Einstein, and Curie was mind-boggling, and I became intrigued. I began to wonder who else had been awarded the prize in chemistry or physics. The next Nobel Prize winner I learned about surfaced in history class during discussions about World War II, which had ended just twelve years prior. We were taught that many of our American soldiers died not from the gunshot wounds themselves but from the fatal infections that set in on the battlefields because of the wounds. I recall our teacher telling us that Professor Alexander Fleming had won the Nobel Prize in Physiology or Medicine for his discovery of penicillin. She said that the discovery of penicillin was the result of an accident in Fleming's laboratory, but no further explanation was given. The teacher focused more on the widespread production and use of penicillin on the battlefields to save lives and how it was a turning point in the war for us and our allies.

Since I was more interested in chemistry and biology than history at the time, I went to the library to learn more about how a revolutionary drug like penicillin could have been discovered by accident. I found out that the culprit was a dirty laboratory benchtop left unattended, resulting in the development of mold near the test tubes and plates that were being used to grow bacteria for study. Fleming noticed that the bacteria immediately adjacent to the mold were dead, whereas the bacteria farther away had survived and were still growing. The mold was analyzed for the possible presence of an antibacterial compound, and that's how penicillin was discovered for the first time.

And so, by age sixteen, I was aware of four powerful examples of what type of discovery it takes to be recognized with the Nobel Prize. I was convinced: experimentation is what it's all about. What if the glassware with the contaminating mold simply had been discarded? How much longer would it have taken before penicillin was discovered? Would it have altered the outcome of World War II?

Around this same time, I wondered why many people lived long and healthy lives, whereas many others developed high blood pressure, diabetes, and suffered strokes and heart attacks. Growing up, I noticed that several of the adults around me were living healthy lives, with no signs of cardiovascular impairment, well into their eighties and nineties. On the other hand, a nearly equal number of adults I knew had developed high blood pressure or experienced a stroke when they were only about fifty or sixty years old. Others had suffered from myocardial infarctions (heart attacks) at relatively young ages.

In most cases, these cardiovascular problems did not appear to run in the family. That is, they appeared not to be hereditary or genetic in origin. It occurred to me that perhaps healthy people produced a molecule that protected their cardiovascular system against injury, whereas unhealthy people produced less or none of this molecule. I had no idea what this molecule might be, if it existed at all, but I hoped that in the future, I would be able to do basic research to study this problem.

To accomplish this, I knew I would have to go to college and graduate school. My growing understanding of chemistry and biology midway through high school convinced me that I would have no difficulty with these subjects in college and beyond. But the question that kept popping up in my mind was whether my high school grades would be good enough to get accepted to a decent school. Despite my straight-A grades in all the mathematics and science classes, my grades in English and social studies were terrible, consisting mostly of C's and one D. I had less than two years to pull up my grades. I would have to ace all classes right up to graduation. The depressing and frightful thought of not being able to study chemistry and biology in college was all the inspiration and motivation I needed to get my act together.

By the end of my third year in high school, I had become a competent enough mechanic that I could rebuild an entire engine and tune it up myself. The main source of my frustration was that I could not legally drive what I had built to race.

When I reached my senior year, my dad surprised me with the news that he wanted to buy me a new car. We went together to the local Ford dealership and ordered a brand-new 1958 Ford Fairlane 500 with the newly designed Interceptor V8 engine. The Interceptor V8 was more expensive than an ordinary engine, so my dad asked me why I wanted it. Luckily, he did not know anything about horsepower or fast cars, so I managed to convince him to get it for me without telling him that Ford had built the Fairlane 500 to compete with the Chevy Impala V8 powerhouse.

After some (legal) modifications and registering my car with track officials, I was ready for my first race.

Now, it was do or die. I pulled up to the starting line in the right lane, and in the left lane came a mean-looking 1958 black Chevy Impala. I was keenly aware that no A-Stock Ford had ever beaten an A-Stock Chevy at Westhampton before. I was nervous, and I could feel my heart pounding. Even my legs were shaking.

But I knew I could beat him as long as I did not spin out of control at the starting line.

The flagman got ready, gave each of us the thumbs-up, and then flagged us off. We both came out of the gate quickly and with no significant wheel spinning. First, I pulled ahead of the Chevy, but he quickly passed me. Then, my engine did what it was intended to do, and I pulled ahead and beat him to the finish line by two car-lengths.

My first drag race had been an exhilarating success! When I returned to the pits in back of the starting line to collect my trophy, I was told that I set a new A-Stock class record of 93 mph. They were proud to have me as a member of the club, and I was so thankful for the opportunity to work with them for a couple of years leading up to this special day. This was a good day indeed.

When I got home from the track, I burst into the living room to show Mom and Dad my Westhampton Raceway Trophy. It wasn't until I held up the trophy in front of them that I realized my mistake. Neither one had known I was even drag racing.

Dad said nothing. Mom, on the other hand, had a lot to say.

"First, it's the damn chemistry set, and now it's drag racing! What am I going to do with you?" she screamed. I calmed her down a bit by explaining the safety of the racetrack with all its rules.

An hour later, Dad asked to see the trophy. I showed it to him. It was about fourteen inches in height and was fixed on a stained block of wood that held a bronze plaque with the inscription "Westhampton Raceway Drag Racing A-Stock Class Record."

He took hold of the trophy and smiled. I could see that he was proud of my accomplishments. But he did not tell me so. At the time, I suspected he was not convinced that this new hobby of mine was a good idea. They were aware that I was hanging around with the guys and working on cars, but racing my own car had come as a surprise. I had not told either of my parents that I had modified my car for drag racing, and I certainly had never mentioned my intention to race it.

One morning, a few days later, while I was in my bedroom reading, my dad walked in and asked me what I was doing. I told him that I was reading up on my favorite subject, chemistry.

"You really like that stuff, don't you? You have been interested in chemicals since you were a kid."

"Yes," I said. "And I plan to go to college to learn much more."

After a brief but genuine smile, Dad changed the subject and got serious.

"About racing the car," he said. "Your mamma is not happy. She is upset and came crying to me this morning. She said that racing cars is dangerous, and you could be hurt."

"But the racetrack is very safe. No accidents ever happen there …"

He interrupted me, "Please do not argue with Mom about this. Give her some time, and she will calm down."

"Okay," I agreed.

Dad got up to leave my room, and when he got to the door, he turned to me. "Congratulations," he said. "Keep up the good work and be safe."

Two months and six trophies later, Dad built me a beautiful trophy case made of Philippine mahogany, the highest quality wood for cabinets and furniture. He then went on to build a much larger trophy case for the club, which had collected over three dozen trophies. What an incredible father I had!

Although I still had a passion for chemistry and biology, the idea of being a race car mechanic and driver also excited me.

With this knowledge and a bit more experience, I reasoned, or perhaps fantasized, that I could eventually open my own speed shop and draw lots of customers. In addition, I could build my own car for drag racing and keep it perfectly tuned for use at the track. I had even found a potential location for my shop on Sunrise Highway in Valley Steam—ideal because on the next block were both an auto racing parts store and an engine milling plant.

Just as I was beginning to convince myself that this was indeed a great idea, I told my dad that I could not decide whether I wanted to be a race car mechanic or go to college and study chemistry. Upon hearing this, Dad stared at me and told me quietly but with conviction that I was not going to be a mechanic or drive race cars for a living. "You are going to college," he said. "You are going to be somebody special."

Chapter 4:
College Bound

When I began to consider attending college, I had no idea yet which profession I would pursue. The only thought in my mind was to learn more chemistry and biology. My intent was to develop a deep enough knowledge base to answer one important question that had persisted in my mind for a long while: is there a molecule we produce that keeps our cardiovascular system healthy?

The only way to find out was to do basic biomedical research in this area. I was an ardent believer in experimentation to advance our knowledge of science. In every facet of my life through both elementary and high school, I used scientific experimentation to advance my knowledge of nearly everything. I clearly saw that understanding what causes heart attacks and strokes was a field in medicine that needed a lot more investigation, since the causes were completely unknown at the time. With proper training, I believed that I would succeed in becoming a competent scientist.

But I knew that to accomplish this, I had to go to college and beyond.

After researching colleges, I concluded midway through my junior year in high school that Columbia University in New York City was perfect because of their excellent programs in chemistry and the biomedical sciences, plus it was an easy commute from Long Beach. But upon sharing my views with my high school advisor, he told me straightaway that I should not get my hopes up because I most likely would not get accepted to Columbia.

"Why not?" I asked. "I've gotten straight A's in all of my science and math courses in high school."

"Yes, but you've gotten straight C's in all of your other courses except for English, in which you got a D last year." Based on that, he advised me instead to apply to a local state college in Long Island.

I was disappointed and heartbroken after hearing my advisor's assessment of my prospects. I could not sleep for days because of his discouraging advice. It seemed to me that my advisor failed to appreciate my passion and expertise in the sciences. He just didn't understand what science meant to me. I guess he was being honest about my poor chances of acceptance to such a competitive university as Columbia because of my terrible grades in the non-sciences. But, I thought, he could have at least recommended a course of action to improve those grades. For instance, that I take extra courses in non-science subjects during the summer months. But he did none of that. His advice was to forget about

Columbia. However, I was not about to take no for an answer. It was never in my nature to give up.

From that moment on, I focused on my English and history classes and, as a result, I brought my grades up to A's in those subjects. In my senior year, once again, I focused on English and history. In the 1950s, the state of New York issued standardized exams, termed State Regents Exams, where a common exam had to be taken by all seniors in all high schools in New York. These standardized exams were only for English and history. Despite my poor grades in these two subjects in the first part of my high school education, I earned A's in my State Regents Exams. In fact, I was in the 96th percentile in English, which surprised the hell out of my English teacher, and me too, for that matter.

Halfway through my senior year, I took a chance and applied for admission to Columbia College in New York City. Columbia had various schools that one could apply to. I chose to major in chemistry and pharmacy, not because I wanted to become a pharmacist but rather because such an education would provide me with the knowledge and background I desired not only in chemistry, but in biology too.

Three months later, a letter came to me in the mail. With a heart rate of over one hundred, I opened the envelope and read the letter. No decision had been made. Instead, I was asked to come in for an interview.

Okay, I thought, *at least it wasn't an outright rejection.* I had three weeks to prepare for my interview. I kept asking myself, *What are they going to ask me? They probably won't ask me about my straight A's in science subjects. It's probably going to be about my C and D grades in non-science.* I had to think of a good answer to such a question.

The interview day arrived. After several anxious moments sitting in a waiting office, a scholarly looking man who appeared to be about sixty years of age called me into the interview. He introduced himself as Professor Samuel Lieberman and then proceeded to tell me that he was an inorganic chemist teaching qualitative and quantitative analysis at the university.

"I see you did very well in all of your science subjects in high school and even worked with Professor Linus Pauling to develop a general chemistry laboratory course as well."

"Yes, sir," I replied.

"I also notice that you did not do as well in English and history," he said. "What's your explanation for that?"

I knew that my explanation had to be both convincing and emotionally stirring. Otherwise, I would have a long and sad train ride home. I explained how my mom and dad were immigrants from Italy and spoke no English until I started grade school. This served as a serious handicap since they could not help me with my homework or anything else related to learning. I had to struggle on my own to do the best I could in grade school and even high school.

"But then how was it possible for you to score straight A's in science and mathematics?" he asked.

I told him that those subjects came naturally to me and that I was easily able to study and learn all the material on my own by reading lots of books. Continuing, I asked him to look at my senior year grades in high school, particularly English and history, and also to note my scores on the New York State Regents exams in these subjects.

Professor Lieberman said, "I know, I know. You made a dramatic improvement. Why did you suddenly make up your mind to accomplish that?"

"My high school advisor had warned me that I would never be accepted into Columbia because of my lousy grades in non-science subjects," I said. "I just had to try to get into Columbia because of my passion for learning more chemistry and biology, so I studied harder than ever before to improve my non-science grades."

"And in so doing, you raised your C and D grades to A's and scored in the 96th percentile in New York State," he said. "Excuse me for a couple of minutes."

He left me sitting alone and walked into another office close by. Two minutes felt like two weeks. He finally returned holding some papers. "Read this and then sign at the bottom of the page if you agree."

My hands trembling, I read the brief document and then looked up at him. "Oh my God, thanks so very much, sir."

The document read something like: "Thank you for applying to the Freshman Class at Columbia University of New York. It is my pleasure to inform you that you have been accepted into the entering class. Please follow the instructions …"

I was ecstatic.

After taking care of the required paperwork, I alternated walking and running to the subway stop and took the line to Penn Station. I was so relieved; I suddenly developed a serious craving for a Nedick's hot dog and an orange drink. This hot dog stand was a unique and popular establishment in Penn Station. Originally known for making and selling a signature orange drink, it had added coffee and donuts to its simple menu, and later hot dogs with a unique mustard relish in a toasted bun. Boy, was that good!

My train ride home was the most relaxing ride of my life. In fact, I fell asleep and had to be awakened as we pulled into the Long Beach station, which, luckily, was the final stop of that Long Island line.

I ran all the way home, entered the house, and screamed. My dad was still at work, but my mom got scared and asked me what was wrong. I grabbed her and gave her a big hug and explained the outcome of my visit to New York City.

"I told you that you would get accepted, didn't I?" Mom said. We both laughed.

"Wait until your father gets home; he's going to be so proud of his son!"

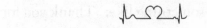

Although I found my first year at Columbia difficult, I did well, and I could easily see myself making it to graduation in four years. My studies focused on chemistry and pharmaceutical sciences. Although I had no intention of practicing pharmacy, I wanted a strong background in chemistry and medicinal chemistry. In particular, I was attracted to all laboratory courses. Indeed, I had been looking forward to working in the lab for several years.

During my undergraduate years at Columbia, my passion for chemistry and biology grew. One of my favorite courses was pharmacology, which is the study of the interactions between chemical molecules and living cells. It combined my love for chemistry and biology, as understanding the chemistry of drug molecules was essential to appreciate how they interact with cells and tissues. I was also particularly drawn to the chemistry courses involving precise laboratory work. One good example was our course in quantitative analysis. Exceedingly demanding, this was the single most-feared course at Columbia, but it turned out to be my favorite. I've always enjoyed working with my hands and handling delicate instruments. Quant, as we called it, demanded that every part of each experimental analysis be conducted with extreme accuracy and precision.

By my senior year at Columbia, I knew that I wanted to pursue basic research in chemistry and biology as a profession. Perhaps such a focus would help me understand the biochemistry of healthy aging. The one discipline that combined these two subject areas was pharmacology.

The University of Wisconsin in Madison had an excellent Department of Pharmacology. And so, I applied for admission and was accepted to their PhD program. One month before I was scheduled to leave, I received a disconcerting letter stating that, due to a disagreement with the dean of the Medical School, the Pharmacology Department chair had decided to leave Wisconsin and quickly drum up a deal with the medical school in Minneapolis. He announced that he would be moving the entire department to the University of Minnesota within a few weeks, and I was to join the department in Minneapolis.

Admittedly, suddenly learning that I was going to Minneapolis instead of Madison caught me off guard. But I had applied to Wisconsin because the Department of Pharmacology was considered to be one of the best in the country. And this was not likely to change despite the new location a few hundred miles north.

I packed my car to the brim with clothes, books, and a few snacks for the 1,200-mile journey from Long Beach to Minneapolis. But instead of heading straight there, I decided to take a slight detour to visit Niagara Falls in Buffalo. I had never been there and seized the opportunity to spend a few hours admiring one of the wonders of our beautiful country. I suspected that this brief moment of serenity might be the last one for quite some time.

PART II:
The Science

"I find that the harder I work, the more luck I seem to have."
— *Thomas Jefferson*

PART II.

Chapter 5:

Graduate School and Basic Research

I spent the next four years in Minneapolis at the University of Minnesota, where I earned a degree of PhD in Pharmacology. Quite often throughout my career, when I tell people that I am a pharmacologist, they respond by asking me where my pharmacy is located. I've had to explain that a pharmacologist is different from a pharmacist. Pharmacists are trained to fill prescriptions, dispense drugs, and be knowledgeable about all drugs they dispense. Pharmacologists also work with drugs and chemicals but in a different way. The life of a typical pharmacologist is one of basic research, conducted either at an academic institution or at a pharmaceutical or biotech company.

The sudden move of the entire Department of Pharmacology from Madison to Minneapolis turned out to be a great experience for me and the other graduate students, as we got to build the department laboratories from scratch. That is, in addition to taking classes and starting our research training, we had to work like carpenters, painters, electricians, furniture haulers, and designers to put together a functioning department as soon as possible.

Combining our efforts, we were able to accomplish this seemingly impossible task within four months. When we finished on Christmas Eve, I was tired, very tired.

$$\sim\!\!\sqrt{2}\!\!\sim$$

Shortly after returning to Minneapolis after the holiday break, I learned that the School of Medicine and the Graduate Schools in the Biomedical Sciences had gotten together and established a special Combined Medical/Graduate Program. This new program allowed students to complete the requirements for both the MD and PhD degrees together in six years instead of eight years, which would be the case if one obtained the MD and PhD separately. I decided to enter the combined program, not because I had any desire to practice medicine but rather to expand my horizons and enlarge my knowledge base to include medicine and pathology so I might be in a more creative position to focus on existing medical problems.

$$\sim\!\!\sqrt{2}\!\!\sim$$

In medical school, I found the courses in gross anatomy, neuroanatomy, embryology, and pathology enjoyable, and everything was fine until I encountered my first interaction with a motorcycle accident victim. The person was rushed to the emergency room with multiple lacerations and contusions. The sight of the free-flowing blood and broken bones had an effect on me that I was never able to overcome. It was clear that the sight of human blood and exposed body parts was not for me. Accordingly, I completed my medical courses and then decided to stick to basic research. There was no way I would ever be able to work with injured patients. In retrospect, I made the correct decision.

In addition to my major in pharmacology, I took courses in cardiovascular physiology, which became my minor. Moreover, since my PhD dissertation research demanded more knowledge in biochemistry, I took several additional courses in biochemistry, including enzymology, energetics, and protein biochemistry. One of the most exciting but difficult graduate-level courses was enzymology, which is essentially a mathematical analysis of the mechanisms by which enzyme proteins catalyze the conversion of one substance to another. This course was taught by Dr. Paul Boyer, a professor in the Department of Biochemistry.

I enjoyed the course because Professor Boyer used a chemical approach to teaching enzymology and protein-protein interactions. He was a superb teacher who delivered each lecture with unusual clarity. Each morning, he would walk into the lecture hall with the posture of a trained soldier, standing perfectly upright for the duration of the entire lecture. He never walked into the classroom with any notes. He proceeded directly to the chalkboard, grabbed a piece of chalk, and held on to it for the entire lecture. There were no handouts of any kind. What he wrote on the board, we wrote down in our notebooks. His lecturing skills were so good that I didn't have any difficulty keeping up, though Professor Boyer repeatedly emphasized that it was essential that we read the textbook assigned to the class.

Boyer was the first professor to make me realize that thinking could be painful. What made this enzymology course so difficult, despite his teaching skills, were his exams. In the first lecture of class, Boyer told us that there would be only two exams: a midterm exam and a final. He had warned us that his exams were fair but not easy and that we needed to prepare thoroughly by using his class notes as a guide in studying from our enzymology textbook. He wrote the most difficult exams I had ever taken.

After the midterm, our graded exams were placed in our graduate department mailboxes. With trembling hands, I managed to open my large envelope. I looked at the top of the page and saw the grade. Boyer had written in bold, blue ink, "70% correct, A-, Good Work."

I didn't know what to think. Seventy percent was a terrible grade, in my book. What did the A-minus signify? He had written, "Good Work." But I wondered how 70 percent correct could be considered "good work." I made an appointment to visit Professor Boyer and ask him to explain the grade to me.

He explained that the 70 percent correct signified that I had gotten 30 percent incorrect. I said to him, "That's quite logical, sir, but what does the A-minus grade mean?"

"Mr. Ignarro, you got the second highest grade in the class of forty students. That deserves an A-minus." He went on. "Your correct answers were very good. Very good. Your understanding of enzyme kinetics, especially the Michaelis-Menten relationship, is noteworthy. Don't worry about the 30 percent incorrect answers. I did not expect anyone to get those correct, and no one did."

As a direct result of my time and effort in learning the basics of enzymology, I was able to apply these principles to the characterization of enzyme proteins later in my research projects. Professor Boyer turned out to be an important influence on my research career going forward. In addition, I remembered his style of teaching and hoped that I might someday be able to communicate with my students in the same way.

Early on in my graduate studies, I began to think again about the question that had captured my attention back in high school: Why do so many adults die from cardiovascular disease, whereas an equal number go on to live healthy, active lives?

With new information, I began to put some of the puzzle pieces together. A healthy lifestyle of eating well and adequate physical activity meant little or no cardiovascular disease. Yet again, my question was *why?* At the time, no one knew the answer to this basic question. Several years after receiving my PhD degree and completing my postdoctoral training at the National Institutes of Health, I'd narrowed my focus to one single question: *Is it possible that at least some of the healthy individuals produce a chemical or molecule in their bodies that protects them against cardiovascular disease, whereas the less lucky individuals produce much less of such a molecule?*

Related thoughts also entered my mind. *Did being overweight or obese trigger a slowdown in the production of this magic molecule? Did living a prolonged sedentary lifestyle also depress the production of the same molecule?* It appeared clear to me that combining the two poor lifestyle habits might exacerbate the problem. At this point, I was hoping to steer my scientific career in a direction that would enable me to answer the question of the chemistry of prolonged health and longevity—what molecule(s) could be responsible for keeping us healthy and ensuring longevity?

When I began graduate school, my mentor, Professor Frederick Shideman, wanted me to study the development of the autonomic nervous system in the embryonic chick heart. Professor Shideman was also the chairman of the Department of Pharmacology. He was interested in understanding the early influence of nerves on heart function and wanted me to start this project so I could determine whether I wanted to continue the project for my PhD thesis dissertation. The nerves that attach to the heart release chemical molecules known as catecholamines, which then stimulate the heart to beat faster and stronger. We wanted to know if attachment of the nerves to the heart was necessary for such nerves to produce and release catecholamines. Although it was fairly difficult research, I enjoyed it because the experiments were working, and I felt like I was making appreciable progress.

The most difficult and frustrating aspect of the research project was the vanishingly small size of some of the embryonic chick hearts. For example, in many cases, I had to use a microscope to dissect the heart from a three-day-old chick embryo. Such hearts were about the size of a single grain of table salt. In order to obtain a sample size large enough to analyze, I had to accumulate about a hundred individual hearts and pool them together.

During my third year, my basic research project had been progressing very well. I had been spending ten hours, every day, working in my lab. On many occasions, I went into the lab on weekends as well. In the summer of 1965, my parents and brother drove from New York to Minneapolis to spend a week with me. This was an exciting visit because I missed seeing my family regularly. Since I was in medical school, my dad wanted to see the hospital and meet some of my patients.

My brother, Angelo, explained to him that I was not training to be that kind of doctor.

Dad responded with, "What do you mean? What kind of doctor does not have patients?"

I cut in and explained that some doctors do important medical research in the laboratory rather than see patients. Dad paused for a moment and then asked to see my laboratory.

The next morning, I drove them to Millard Hall, the building housing my lab. As most of the buildings were locked on Sundays, I took out my keys to open three different sets of doors to reach my lab. I could see that Dad was quite impressed by my having keys to unlock such an enormous building in a medical center. Finally, we made it to my lab and walked inside. Both my mom and dad stood there with their mouths agape, staring at all of the laboratory equipment and supplies.

Later that evening, over dinner, I asked my parents if they had any questions about my training. Dad noted that the walls needed to be cleaned and painted and that the laboratory tabletops should be replaced with new ones. That was the painter and carpenter emerging from my father.

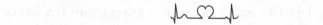

My tenure at the University of Minnesota lasted exactly four years, the basic research took me about three years to complete. My basic research accomplishments in graduate school were good enough to publish my cardiovascular work in top, peer-reviewed medical journals. I had enough data to write four separate research papers for publication. In working with Professor Shideman, he suggested that we submit the work as four back-to-back papers in the *Journal of Pharmacology and Experimental Therapeutics*. I questioned his suggestion because there had never before been four back-to-back papers by the same group of authors published in this prestigious journal. I was preparing myself for a quick letter of rejection from the journal's editor-in-chief. But instead, in 1968, all four papers were accepted for publication, a record that still stands to this day.

The next step was to find a suitable laboratory in which to execute meaningful postdoctoral basic research. Getting a PhD degree alone is not sufficient for landing a good academic or industrial job. One must engage in an independent research program away from any mentors in graduate school. The idea is to prove that you're capable of "independent" research. That's where a postdoctoral fellowship comes in.

I knew exactly where I wanted to do my postdoctoral training. The laboratory had to be a pharmacology lab with a chemistry approach to answer important questions in pharmacology and physiology. The National Institutes of Health (NIH) in Bethesda, Maryland, housed many different Institutes, each focusing on a given aspect of human disease. I was interested in cardiovascular disease, so the National Heart, Lung, and Blood Institute (NHLBI) was for me. Then came the icing on the cake. The NHLBI established the Laboratory of Chemical Pharmacology (LCP) for those interested in pursuing a chemical approach to pharmacology research. It was such a perfect fit; it seemed the LCP was created just for me. I applied, was accepted into the program, and started in September of 1966, a few months after obtaining my PhD from the University of Minnesota.

The NIH was a truly spectacular place to conduct research for multiple reasons. The resources including funds, supplies, and instrumentation were seemingly endless. Another important reason, at least for me, was that so many of the best scientists in the world had positions at the NIH. A constant flow of lectures were given by in-house scientists as well as those invited from outside NIH. Moreover, the NIH offered courses in so many different areas of biology and medicine, and anyone could attend any course provided they had the time. But I took advantage of another opportunity, namely, to walk into a few other laboratories and introduce myself to those who directed the basic research.

Several labs at the NIH focused their work in areas that were also of great interest to me. I figured that witnessing such work would help me to plan and perform my own research. That's essentially what I did in graduate school when I needed to learn and develop new methodologies for my work. I learned not to be shy in approaching others, but at the same time, not to be excessively self-assertive.

The first scientist I looked for, about a month after I started at the NIH, was Dr. Julius Axelrod. I had employed several of his original assay techniques in my graduate studies, and I wanted to introduce myself. As I walked into his lab, I immediately recognized him. Dr. Axelrod was easy to spot because he was a short gentleman who wore a patch over one eye, which he had lost as a result of an accident in a chemistry laboratory.

He was busy chatting with one of his fellows as I entered. Several minutes later, as he started walking toward the lab door, he spotted me.

"May I help you?" he asked.

"Yes," I said. "My name is Lou Ignarro, and I've just started my postdoctoral position with Dr. Elwood Titus in the Laboratory of Chemical Pharmacology. My mentor in graduate school was

Professor Fred Shideman, and he told me to give you his warmest regards."

"Thank you very much," Dr. Axelrod replied with a grin. "Now I know who you are! You just published four back-to-back papers in the *Journal of Pharmacology and Experimental Therapeutics* on catecholamines in the developing embryonic heart." He stepped forward and welcomed me with a beaming smile and a warm handshake. "Great work!"

He placed his hand on the back of my shoulder and asked me to walk with him through one of his laboratories. He went on: "I noticed that you used several technological methods that were developed right here in my laboratory."

"I could never have completed my research had it not been for your published methods," I said. "I am delighted to learn that you recalled my four publications."

"What kind of research will you be doing here at the NIH? Can I be of any further assistance?"

"Yes, as a matter of fact. Although I am engaged in a somewhat different research project in someone else's laboratory here at the NIH, I really enjoyed my graduate work on catecholamines in the heart, and I want to keep up with developments in this field. Moreover, I may be able to use some of your methods again, this time in my research here at the NIH. You are the world's expert on catecholamines, and I would like to know if it's okay for me to step into your lab every now and then to see what's going on."

"My lab is your lab. Anytime you want to play." He went on to offer me some lab bench space in the corner if I wanted to conduct a side project with him and his fellows.

I took him up on his offer and visited his lab every week for a few hours. However, I did not have the time to engage in a separate project in his lab because I was committed to my own research efforts in my assigned laboratory with Dr. Elwood Titus. Instead, I used my frequent visits to attend Dr. Axelrod's weekly laboratory meetings to learn more about specific aspects of cardiovascular pharmacology.

The focus of my basic research in graduate school was cardiovascular pharmacology and physiology. At the NIH, my focus was more on taking a chemical approach to better our understanding of cardiovascular pharmacology and physiology. But the key was my passion for the "cardiovascular" field. I truly believed that Dr. Axelrod's laboratory approaches could afford me the opportunity to strengthen my own research program, and I did not want to miss out on this unique opportunity.

Dr. Axelrod (or Julie, as everyone called him) loved working with young investigators. For example, he always told us that if we thought we had a good idea, we should pursue it until we either validated it or showed clearly that it was not such a good idea after all. His attitude motivated and inspired me.

He was a good and humble man, liked by all. Learning good experimental procedures was not the only thing I took away from his lab. I had developed a genuine admiration for the way he treated his research personnel and motivated them to perform to the best of their abilities. Another important asset gained from my interaction with Axelrod's group was the importance of conducting weekly lab meetings involving everyone working in the lab. This kept everyone organized and in tune along the same path to attain the goals of the research projects. In thinking ahead a few years, I knew the day would come when I would be confronted with the responsibility of directing my own laboratory research group. I hoped that I would be able to use Dr. Axelrod's model in establishing my basic research group.

Two years after I completed my postdoctoral fellowship at the NIH, I was delighted and ecstatic to learn that Julius Axelrod was awarded the 1970 Nobel Prize in Physiology or Medicine.

Dr. Axelrod wasn't the only important person I met while living in the Washington, DC, area. One Saturday evening, an NIH colleague and I went to a government-sponsored dance in Georgetown. The organization was termed the Junior Officers and Professionals Association, and the dance was referred to as the JOPA party. This was a weekly dance open to any government employee wishing to attend and mingle with about three hundred people. Working at the NIH, I met these qualifications. I had never been to such a gathering, and I enjoyed the international flavor of the event. After all, this was Washington, DC. As I walked through the dense dancing crowd, I spotted a young lady standing in the corner, talking with two others. I approached her and asked if she would like to dance with me. After pausing for a few moments, she agreed.

While dancing, I learned her name was Jan, and we began a dialogue. She was one of several executive secretarial assistants for the postmaster general. In addition, she shared that she had previously worked in the West Wing of the White House, first for President Kennedy and then for President Johnson, after Kennedy's assassination. In the middle of our conversation, I asked her for a second dance, but she turned me down. Jan said she wanted to spend some time with her girlfriends, whom she hadn't seen in weeks.

Just before the dance party ended, Jan came over to me and said she enjoyed chatting with me and that perhaps we might run into each other again at a future JOPA party. *That was unexpected*, I thought, but it left the door open for a future get-together. As I had not dated much in graduate school due to my workload, I was eager to see her again. She was intelligent, witty, and held a responsible position in the government.

Although I was busy with my research at the NIH, I decided that all work and no play was not what the doctor ordered. I looked forward to my free Saturday nights, especially at the JOPA parties.

Eventually, I ran into Jan again. This time, she was standing in the corner by herself. Without delay, I approached her and asked her to dance with me. She agreed, and we danced and chatted all evening long.

We started dating a few weeks later and saw each other no more frequently than once a week for months. I explained to Jan that my basic research was important to me and that I simply did not have the time to go out more frequently. Often, however, we would spend the entire Saturday or Sunday together before going out for the evening. The most common topic for discussion was her desire to quit work to enter into a training program to become a Catholic nun. Jan was a very religious Greek Orthodox. And I had not been to church in over ten years.

Despite this big difference, we got along very well and fell in love. *What now*, I thought? Jan said that she would continue to see me for about a month or so, but then she would stop and make plans to leave Washington, DC. I spent the next month, on a daily basis, trying to convince her not to leave the area and to remain here with me.

Finally, she said to me, "Lou, if I stay, would you marry me?"

I paused for a very long minute. "Maybe."

"Well, when you decide one way or the other, please do let me know. But I plan to hand in my resignation to the postmaster general in two weeks."

That clearly meant I had two weeks to make up my mind. At that point, I was not certain what I wanted to do. Did I want to commit to such a "permanent" relationship? Jan was a devout and God-fearing Catholic, whereas I was just Catholic by birth. If we got married and things didn't work out, how could I ever think about divorce? The marriage would be permanent!

I didn't have enough time to reason this out. I did not want to lose Jan. Moreover, I was lonely, being buried in my work. I needed to make up my mind now.

I picked up the phone and called Jan. "I would like to see you right away," I said. The next evening, I asked her to marry me.

We were married a few months later, in October of 1967, in a Greek Orthodox church in Arlington, Virginia. The next morning, we boarded a flight to the Bahamas for our honeymoon. That was the first full week of total relaxation that I had enjoyed in a very long time.

Chapter 6:
My Early Career in the Drug Industry

B y the end of 1968, I was a bona fide chemical pharmacologist. After completing a postdoctoral fellowship, my original intention was to apply for a starting instructor position at a university, but I was convinced to take an alternate path.

A large pharmaceutical company (Geigy, later known as Ciba-Geigy, and later yet took on the name Novartis) approached me and offered me a job. In our conversation, they told me that my role would be to join the team of biologists and chemists who were responsible for drug discovery in the field of inflammation and arthritis. I was a bit concerned because my expertise up to that point had been in the cardiovascular area, and I was skeptical about trying something new. However, they argued that based on the success of my basic research in graduate school and at the NIH, they believed I would be successful. Then I recalled a quote from Albert Einstein, "A person who never made a mistake never tried anything new."

I accepted the position at Geigy's headquarters in Ardsley, New York, a scenic small town just north of the Bronx. Moreover, Geigy was only an hour's drive to my parents. This would give me the opportunity to see them fairly frequently on weekends. Although my mom was still relatively young, my dad was about seventy-two years old at the time, and I wanted to be with him as often as I could. However, despite his age, he was in better shape than most men in their fifties. He still worked six days a week as a carpenter and was in excellent health. Nevertheless, I had missed seeing him during my years in Minneapolis. Now, I would have the chance to be with him several times each month.

Jan was looking forward to moving to the New York City area for a change in scenery and weather. We moved into a spacious apartment in White Plains, which was only a ten-mile drive to Ardsley. Jan had made the decision not to pursue a job in New York because she wanted to have children and raise a family. Reluctantly, I said that was fine. I had hoped she would work at least until she got pregnant because we were financially burdened as I started my position at Geigy. But after several months of salary, it turned out to be more than manageable.

The company was generous and flexible. For example, in addition to my well-defined role in drug discovery, I was permitted to conduct a limited amount of basic research that was unrelated to drug discovery. This opportunity gave me the chance to study certain areas in pharmacology that were of great interest to me but unrelated to the development of anti-inflammatory drugs.

This turned out to be instrumental to my growth in the field of basic research.

During the early months of my new adventure in the drug industry, one of my colleagues at work introduced me to Dr. Paul Greengard, who had been a neuroscientist and chairman of the Department of Biochemistry at Geigy Pharmaceuticals just before I started working there. His role had been to direct his knowledge in biochemistry to drug discovery. He invited me to lunch and wanted to know where I'd done my graduate training. After I told him about my training in chemical pharmacology at the NIH, he asked why I'd elected to go to the drug industry rather than academia, to which I replied, "Well, Dr. Greengard, they offered me a job that I could not refuse."

After he insisted that I call him Paul, he asked, "What do you mean by they offered you a job you could not refuse? What does that mean?"

"Well, the salary is double what I'd be paid in academia, and my role is to serve as one of three directors of the drug discovery program for anti-inflammatory drugs ..."

He interrupted me with a booming voice. "Will Geigy allow you to engage in any publishable basic research unrelated to any drug discovery agenda?"

His loud pitch surprised me, and it was evident that he was trying to raise a very important point.

"Yes, Bill Cash, the chairman of Biochemistry, told me that I would be allowed to do basic research unrelated to drug development."

Greengard raised his arm and pointed a finger at me. "I don't believe that, and you shouldn't either! That's what they told me, too, and it did not work out that way!"

I sat stunned. I didn't know what to say.

"And one more thing," Dr. Greengard said as he wagged his finger three more times. "The salary is not important at your young age, when you are just starting your career in research."

Then he stood up and began walking around in small circles with his head down and said, "On the other hand, what is important is that you develop a basic research program that will command international recognition. You won't be able to do that at Geigy! I promise you."

I felt deflated and dejected, but I understood what he was trying to tell me. I thought that perhaps Bill Cash, Paul's replacement as chair of Biochemistry, would be more lenient and allow me some free time to do my own research. But I could not be certain of that, at least not yet.

He repeated his concerns. "I can tell you, most assuredly, that you will not be able to achieve that goal by working in the drug industry. You've done such outstanding work at Minnesota and the NIH. Why do you want to throw all that away now? You need to get an academic position at a notable university."

"Dr. Greengard—I mean Paul—since I just started at the company, I don't think it would be appropriate for me to simply leave and go to academia."

He stopped walking in circles and looked right at me. His reaction to my statement was noncommittal. He stared at me with no facial expression.

"I think I can learn something by continuing here for a while," I continued. "For example, directing a large program in drug discovery will give me experience in what it takes to get a drug to market …"

Greengard looked into my eyes. His lips tightened, indicating that he did not necessarily agree with my optimistic plan. But then he relaxed somewhat. "Your short-term plan is a reasonable one," he said. "And you can call me any time you have any questions."

I felt a slight sense of relief, so I asked another question. "So, tell me, Paul, why did *you* leave the drug industry for an academic position?"

"Unlike you, the executives at Geigy frowned every time I told them that basic research was essential to novel drug development. I was told that they were not interested in so-called novel drugs. The only drugs they wanted were more of the same existing drugs but more potent and safer. In other words, all they wanted were "me too" drugs. That's not research. They were interested only in sales and didn't care what kind of drugs were developed. That was not for me. And so, I resigned my position."

"Was there any research project in particular that you wanted to pursue?"

"Yes indeed," he said. "A new cyclic nucleotide molecule, cyclic GMP, was discovered in human urine a few years back and has been recently found to exist in the brain. Moreover, enzymes have been discovered that synthesize this molecule in the body ..."

Greengard explained that cyclic AMP had been proven to be exceedingly important in biology as a key intracellular second messenger molecule in mammalian cells, and it stands to reason that the newly discovered cyclic GMP would prove to be biologically important as well.

He went on, "I want to devote my time and effort to understanding the biological significance of cyclic GMP, especially in the brain. I am a neuroscientist, and that's what I want to do."

I was intrigued and left our conversation convinced that he had made an excellent choice to leave the industry and start a research career in academics.

Paul Greengard had left Geigy Pharmaceuticals in 1967, one year before I was recruited, to take an academic position at Yale University, where he could focus his basic research on cyclic GMP and the brain. Ten years later, he joined the faculty at Rockefeller University. He kept telling me at conferences that, if I were smart, I, too, would focus my attention on cyclic GMP.

Paul was so adamant about my getting into cyclic GMP that I spent a few hours in the library to learn more. I learned that this molecule had the properties of a potential signaling molecule inside cells to control cellular function. But nothing more was known. Having nothing to lose, I decided to investigate whether cyclic GMP was important in the inflammatory process, which was my field of drug discovery at Geigy.

In this way, I was able to combine my responsibilities in drug discovery with my insatiable desire to engage in original basic research. I convinced the Geigy executive team that success with this research project might enable my drug discovery team to come up with a new and more effective anti-inflammatory drug. They were happy with my plan, and I was essentially left alone to do my thing. The group making this decision was different from the group that had turned down Greengard's request to do basic research. I was the lucky one, at least at Geigy.

Within two years, my laboratory had demonstrated that cyclic GMP played a key role in modulating lysosomal enzyme release from human neutrophils during inflammation. In other words, we found that cyclic GMP was a signaling molecule in controlling inflammation. This discovery was thanks almost exclusively to Paul Greengard for inspiring me to study cyclic GMP. At about this time, the Nobel Prize was awarded for the discovery of the other cyclic nucleotide, cyclic AMP, to recipient Professor Earl Sutherland from Vanderbilt University. It hadn't yet occurred to me that Paul might be awarded the Nobel Prize. Thirty years later, in the year 2000, Paul Greengard was awarded the Nobel Prize in Physiology or Medicine for his seminal work on signal transduction in the nervous system.

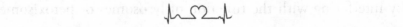

Working on my cyclic GMP project was challenging, exciting, and productive. But I recognized my need to learn more about the inflammatory process to be in the best possible position to develop novel anti-inflammatory drugs. To better prepare myself for this formidable task, I often commuted to nearby Rockefeller University (formerly called the Rockefeller Institute) and Cornell University's downtown Manhattan campus to expand my knowledge of the cell biology and biochemistry of the inflammatory process. On one of my visits, I went to the directory located on the ground level and looked for the name Christian de Duve. I sought him out because of the prominence of his basic research on the inflammatory process in the literature I'd been studying. Professor de Duve had discovered that cells contain two unique organelles (intracellular components) that are involved in mediating inflammation, termed lysosomes and peroxisomes. Lysosomes were so named because these tiny organelles release substances that lyse and kill cells. Peroxisomes release peroxides, which also damage or kill cells. Therefore, both types of organelle can cause inflammation. I thought it reasonable that novel chemical compounds, which could interfere with the release of such inflammatory substances, might prove to be effective anti-inflammatory drugs.

My responsibility in the drug discovery program at Geigy was to come up with an anti-inflammatory drug that worked by mechanisms that are distinct from those for existing drugs on the market. None of the marketed anti-inflammatory drugs worked by interfering with the function of lysosomes or peroxisomes. Here was my opportunity to gear up my laboratory to find such a drug. Perhaps I could learn something from Professor de Duve's research laboratory. Well, there was only one way to find out.

I wandered into Professor de Duve's laboratory and asked someone there if it would be possible to speak with him. The gentleman led me to Professor de Duve's office, right around the corner.

The door was open, and Professor de Duve was seated at his desk, wearing a white lab coat over his white shirt and tie. He looked up from a book he was reading, stood up, and said, "Hello, are you looking for me?"

He was about my height, five feet nine inches, and had a full head of wavy graying hair. He appeared to be in his late fifties and had a distinct smile, which made me feel welcome.

After exchanging a few pleasantries, he asked again if he could help me.

That question was music to my ears. "Professor de Duve," I said, "you most definitely can help me. Is there any way I could observe experiments in your lab from time to time to learn more about the inflammatory process?"

He went on to ask me if I wanted to observe anything in particular. I indicated that I was particularly interested in lysosomes because these organelles contain a variety of proteolytic enzymes that could provoke local inflammation if such lysosomes were discharged from inflammatory cells, such as circulating white blood cells. "I would like to learn how to isolate lysosomes from cells and determine whether anti-inflammatory drugs are capable of somehow preventing lysosomal enzyme release."

"I like your reasoning," he said as he walked me around the corner to his labs. "Welcome to my laboratory."

He proceeded to introduce me to no less than ten of his post-doctoral fellows, visiting professors, and technicians. He told them that I would become a familiar face in the months to come. Admittedly, I did not expect such a warm welcome.

Professor de Duve also informed me that Rockefeller University had several ongoing courses and seminars on cell biology and the inflammatory process and that I was more than welcome to attend. I took him up on both offers and visited Rockefeller University once or twice every month.

Chris de Duve and I quickly became good friends and colleagues. About a year after I started to visit his laboratory, I asked the chairman of the Department of Biochemistry at Geigy Pharmaceuticals to invite Professor de Duve to the company to give a talk on his work in inflammation. Professor de Duve gladly accepted our invitation. He made the forty-five-minute drive from Rockefeller University to Ardsley in his Porsche sports car. When he arrived, I was waiting for him in the parking lot, and I seized the opportunity to take him to my laboratory to show him what we were doing with lysosomes, which he had discovered many years back. De Duve asked me lots of logical questions and had several important suggestions to pursue in my approach to developing novel anti-inflammatory drugs.

In the months to come, I went on to show that certain chemical compounds could stabilize the lysosomal membrane and thereby slow or prevent the release of its contents into the intracellular environment. Such an effect resulted in prevention of inflammation and increased cell survival in laboratory animal models of inflammation and arthritis. We used this assay as a screening tool to select active anti-inflammatory drug candidates from the dozens of chemical substances provided to us from the medicinal chemistry department.

On one of my drives to Rockefeller University, I turned on the radio and tuned into a rock 'n' roll station, and a song I'd never heard captured my attention. I heard the DJ, Casey Kasem, talk about an up-and-coming star who had just released a tune that he predicted would quickly reach the top of the charts. He was referring to Elton John and introduced the tune *Crocodile Rock*. I immediately took to it and became an instant fan.

Listening to the music of Elton John in both my office and research laboratory created an atmosphere conducive to creative thought, as his elegant music was both soothing and uplifting, and it broke the monotony of repetitive laboratory procedures. In the mid-1970s, CD players did not exist. Instead, one of my lab technicians set up a combination radio/record player and neatly wired it to several speakers positioned throughout the lab. Since I was such an ardent fan of Elton John, I purchased all of his hits and kept them in a file in the lab for everyone to play. Although the people in the lab brought in many of their own favorite re-cords, the most frequently played songs were those of Elton John. I often left my office door wide open so the lively tunes drifted into every corner of the lab.

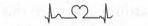

Less than a year after we moved to White Plains, Jan became pregnant. During my first year at Geigy, I was putting in ten-to-twelve-hour working days and even went to the lab on some Saturdays. This was a sticky point for Jan, who frequently questioned why I had to spend so much time at work. She was not a scientist and had no concept of the demands of a basic research career in the biomedical sciences. On some occasions, she expressed her dissatisfaction by refusing to prepare dinner for us. Jan pointed out her concern about my spending such long hours at work once our child was born. I was also concerned and recognized that I would have to change my schedule soon.

Jan made it through her pregnancy with no morning sickness or any other significant discomforts and, on January 10, 1970, spent only a few hours in labor. I had wanted to be present at the delivery, but things had progressed so rapidly that I arrived at the hospital mere minutes after our beautiful daughter, Heather, was born. That was probably for the best, as I'm certain I would have been a nervous wreck had I been present during childbirth.

I stayed at the hospital until the evening and then went home for some much-needed rest. The following day, I returned to the hospital. It was Super Bowl (IV) Sunday, which I had planned to watch at home because my favorite team, the Minnesota Vikings, was playing the Kansas City Chiefs, and the Vikings were highly favored to win.

As it turns out, I was fortunate not to have watched the game because the Vikings, who were two-touchdown favorites, were trounced by the Chiefs. This was the second consecutive year that I was most disappointed with the outcome of the Super Bowl. But none of it mattered as I gently picked up Heather and rocked her to sleep in my arms.

Mom and daughter remained in the hospital for about three days before we all went home together. I took two weeks off from the laboratory to help out at home. Most of my time was spent by Heather's side, even when she was asleep. Jan often found me sleeping on the hardwood floor next to the crib.

After starting back at work, I managed to get things done within an eight-hour day and only five days a week. It was a joy to come home every evening to be at Heather's side. She started to walk by the time she was nine months of age, and she got herself into anything and everything she could reach, including my mustache. At first, she would touch and gently stroke my mustache, but then she quickly caught on to grabbing the whiskers and trying to pluck them one by one. After discovering my mustache, she graduated to pulling my hair. Unfortunately (or fortunately, depending how you look at it), I did not have much hair to pull. Eventually, I taught her to slap the top of my balding head instead of trying to pull out my last remaining hairs.

Although I cut down my hours, my research didn't slow by any stretch of the imagination. During my last two years in the industry, my laboratory had found an interesting chemical compound that demonstrated potent anti-inflammatory and analgesic (pain relieving) activities in several different animal models of inflammation and arthritis. Moreover, this compound of interest displayed remarkable activity in stabilizing lysosomes and preventing the release of inflammatory mediators. The compound was also relatively free of side effects in the animals studied. As these data were consistent with a compound that could go forward in development, I made the recommendation for approval to conduct further studies required to submit an NDA (new drug application) to the FDA (Food and Drug Administration). My recommendation was approved, and various departments within the company were called into action to schedule the compound for further development, which consisted mostly of toxicology or safety studies in animals.

I was especially pleased with the company's decision to move forward in developing this potential drug because I believed that what I had learned from Chris de Duve about inflammation helped me find a novel anti-inflammatory compound with a unique mechanism of action. But after spending two or three years in drug discovery, I came to realize that something was missing. During my doctoral studies, I'd always thought that I would enjoy teaching graduate and medical students. I had no such opportunity in the drug industry. I could do this only in an academic institution. Fueling this desire to teach was the mounting excitement and success of my cyclic GMP work in the laboratory. Despite the success of my anti-inflammatory drug discovery program, I realized it was time to leave the drug industry and begin an academic career in basic research and teaching.

Chapter 7:
My Burning Question

Beyond the game-changing invention of dynamite for industry, one of the most significant scientific/medical discoveries of the nineteenth century was made in Alfred Nobel's factories. First, a pattern was observed that within hours of entering the factories on weekday mornings, many of the workers complained of throbbing headaches, which subsided after working hours. At the same time, factory workers suffering from chest pain, or angina pectoris, due to coronary artery disease or heart failure often experienced dramatic relief during the work week, but the chest pains recurred on weekends.

These observations were eventually brought to the attention of the medical community, but no definitive conclusions were drawn. Physiologists and physicians were determined to unravel the enigma because there was no treatment of angina pectoris at the time.

In the late 1860s, two interesting observations were made. Researchers suspected, and later demonstrated, that the nitroglycerin used to make the dynamite was the culprit of both headaches and anti-anginal effects. Nitroglycerin is a volatile, thick liquid that spewed its vapors into the surrounding air. Anyone working nearby would inhale the nitroglycerin vapors and experience headaches and/or relief of chest pain within minutes. Although researchers were able to conclude that nitroglycerin was responsible for the pronounced pharmacological effects, the mechanism of action was unknown. No one could figure out how nitroglycerin, a powerful explosive, could relieve chest pain in some and cause headaches in others. The suspicion offered by scientists was that nitroglycerin might have vasodilator activity, which would be expressed upon inhalation of its fumes into the lungs and subsequent absorption into the blood circulating through the lungs. At the time, scientists suspected that cerebral artery dilation might bring about severe headaches. Moreover, the chest pain relief suggested that there might also be dilation of the coronary arteries, thereby promoting more blood flow and consequent oxygen delivery to the heart of patients with obstructive coronary blood flow.

About ten years later, in 1879, William Murrell reported that a 1 percent solution of nitroglycerin administered orally to patients with coronary artery disease relieved angina and prevented subsequent attacks. Murrell's team then set out to develop a safe and non-explosive dosage form of nitroglycerin that could be carried and taken by patients. Experimentation by Murrell's team revealed that tiny amounts of nitroglycerin, less than one milligram, could be mixed with certain sugars to stabilize the nitroglycerin, and this mixture brought prompt relief of anginal pain. Accordingly, small tablets of the compressed nitroglycerin/sugar mixture were prepared and tested orally in patients with angina, and the rest is history. Similar nitroglycerin tablets are widely used today.

But one important question remained. What is the mechanism of vasodilator action of the most powerful explosive chemical discovered in the nineteenth century? The answer to this question would not be known for another hundred years.

In January of 1973, I accepted an academic position at Tulane University Medical Center in New Orleans and began my academic career. One important reason I chose Tulane University is that there was a faculty member studying cyclic GMP. I had learned enough about cyclic GMP during my research at Ciba-Geigy to recognize the potential future of this signaling molecule.

Jan, Heather, and I moved to New Orleans to support this career change and settled in Gretna, a suburb on the west bank of the Mississippi. Heather was three years old at the time, and I promised Jan that I would try to take more responsibility in raising my daughter, although I was not quite certain how. Heather was a happy and energetic young girl who quickly made friends with anyone and everyone in the neighborhood. I spent a great deal of time with her on the weekends, taking her to parks and teaching her how to run and play softball and ride a bicycle. And

I loved helping her with her reading, writing, and math skills. I could bond with her over the academics of it all.

New Orleans was a fabulous place to take Heather on adventures through the town and adjacent suburbs. She enjoyed walking through the French Quarter and listening to the jazz music played outdoors on so many corners. This was totally different from the New York suburbs, and she loved it. One of her favorite excursions was to walk through the Lafayette Cemetery in the Garden District. This was the burial grounds for many famous and notable persons of the past two hundred years. But what intrigued Heather was that all tombs were located above the ground, and many were enormous, reaching heights of fifteen or twenty feet. The water table in New Orleans is too high, only one or two feet below the surface, to permit coffins to be buried underground. Instead, the city adopted the Spanish style of vault graves.

Although my young daughter was becoming fascinated with New Orleans, my wife and I were less enchanted. The lifestyle in New Orleans was completely different from what we were used to in New York. We felt that we were living in one big party town that did not even quiet down at night. It was like Mardi Gras every day of the year. The best part of New Orleans was the unique cuisine. The worst part was the abhorrent racism, which we did not know how to deal with. It added additional stress to our lives, and soon, the tension would come to a head.

On October 7, 1974, a Monday, I learned on the evening news that the Nobel Prize in Physiology or Medicine had been awarded to Professor Christian de Duve for his discoveries on the structural and functional organization of the cell. That was the most exciting news I had heard in a while. Having read most of his work as I planned my own research, I firmly believed that he deserved such an accolade. Somehow, I felt connected to Chris and the Nobel Prize, perhaps because I had gotten to know him personally.

The following morning, I called de Duve's office to congratulate him. However, his assistant answered the phone and told me that he was at his other laboratory in Belgium and would return November 1 and that he planned to remain in New York through the Christmas holiday.

I thanked her for her help and immediately took out my calendar. The Thanksgiving holiday weekend, I thought, would be a convenient time to leave my lab in New Orleans and spend a week or so with Mom and Dad in Long Beach, and while I was at it, take the train to Manhattan to visit Chris.

I arrived on a Wednesday, the day before Thanksgiving, and decided to go into Manhattan on the following Monday. As I approached his office, I realized that I had not called in advance to make an appointment or even inquire if he was there. But, as I reached the office, I saw Chris chatting with two other gentlemen.

As one who does not like to interrupt anyone in the middle of a conversation, I paused and waited nearby. As the conversation ended, Chris happened to look my way. He smiled upon seeing me and strode over to me, his hand extended.

"I am so delighted to see you! It's been at least a couple of years. What brings you here?"

I shook his hand. "I wanted to come congratulate you in person for being awarded the Nobel Prize. Of course, I knew it would happen but not when."

He took me into one of his laboratories to see some of his people. Everyone was delighted and proud that Chris had won the Nobel Prize. He invited all of us downstairs to the café for coffee.

I took the opportunity to ask, "Chris, how did you feel when you first learned of the prize?"

He was a humble man and refused to take much credit for his discoveries. He turned to look at his people sitting at the table, lifted both arms up in the air, and said, "It is not I who deserves the prize. Rather it is the people in my laboratory who should receive the prize. They did all the work."

Then he went on to say, "I am delighted that my two close friends share the prize with me. George Palade and Albert Claude certainly deserve such recognition because of their major contributions to cell biology."

"Chris, you, too, are highly worthy of the Nobel Prize. It was you, and you alone, who discovered and coined the names lysosomes, peroxisomes, and autophagy."

"Well, thank you very kindly, Lou," he said.

As we started to head back to his office, he told me, "You picked a good day to visit me because tomorrow, I'll be off to Stockholm for the Nobel Prize festivities."

Chris explained to me that the actual Nobel ceremony would be on December 10, the anniversary of Alfred Nobel's death. He also revealed that he and his fellow Laureates would be giving separate lectures on their work.

I felt that I had taken a lot of his time, and I was ready to leave. After wishing him a safe trip and a spectacular time in Stockholm, I told him that I hoped to see him again in the near future. "Thanks, Lou, for coming all this way to see me," he said. "Good luck with your work on lysosome membrane stabilization by anti-inflammatory drugs."

We shook hands, and he gave me a gentle hug as we said our goodbyes.

The awarding of the Nobel Prize to Professor de Duve had a profound impact on me and my own early basic research career. As a person, I was taken by his humble nature and openness to share his laboratory with me. As a scientist, I was impressed with the logical way he approached science to answer insightful questions about cell biology. I learned a great deal from Chris, and it deepened my appreciation of the significance of the Nobel Prize.

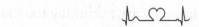

As I continued developing my cyclic GMP research program at Tulane, I learned exciting news about a newly marketed anti-inflammatory drug, and the news made my day. A former colleague of mine at Geigy called me with the spectacular news.

When I was in the drug discovery program at Geigy Pharmaceuticals, my principal responsibility had been to find novel chemical compounds with a unique profile of anti-inflammatory activity that could eventually be tested in clinical trials. More specifically, my drug discovery laboratory was involved in testing several dozen newly synthesized chemicals using a variety of *in vitro* assays, in which known anti-inflammatory drugs were active. Any compounds found to be active in these assays were then tested further, using *in vivo* animal models, such as mice and rats bred to develop inflammation and arthritis. After about four years of testing, we identified three drug candidates for possible clinical trials. One of them was active in stabilizing lysosomal membranes and inhibiting the release of inflammatory enzymes. This was the assay I had learned from Professor de Duve at Rockefeller University. As it turned out, after I left the drug industry for academia, a New Drug Application was filed with the FDA for clinical trials using this particular compound. A few years later, this drug was approved by the FDA and marketed as diclofenac (under the trade name of Voltaren).

In view of my earlier reservations about working in the drug industry, which led me to leave, I wasn't thinking too much about the work I had done at Geigy or what might result from it. And so, the sudden news about diclofenac was unexpected but fabulous. I accomplished what I set out to accomplish. It doesn't get much better than that. At this point, my self-esteem was soaring to new levels.

I couldn't wait to tell two people of the results of my work in the drug industry. One was Paul Greengard, who had urged me to get out of the industry as quickly as possible to start a career in academics before I disappeared into the night. The other was none other than Chris de Duve, who had wished me luck in developing a novel anti-inflammatory drug that worked by stabilizing lysosomes, his favorite organelle.

My basic research program was off to an excellent start and continued to be productive for the twelve-year duration of my tenure at Tulane University. This was my first shot at an academic career, and I knew I would have to perform rigorous work to envision and put together a program to enable me to answer that one persistent question that had captured my attention back in high school: Why is it that only some people develop cardiovascular and related disorders? This question had been in the back of my mind through graduate school, to my PhD, and I'd finally narrowed my focus to one single hypothesis: *Is it possible that at least some of the healthy individuals produce a chemical or molecule in their bodies that protects them against cardiovascular disease, whereas the less lucky individuals produce much less of such a molecule?* Now, at Tulane, I finally had the opportunity to give it my undivided attention.

I'd observed that nearly all of the adults I knew who had developed health problems were significantly overweight and did not appear to be engaging in appreciable physical activity, whereas the healthy ones were a normal weight and active. In my family, on both my dad's side and my mom's, numerous aunts, uncles, and cousins, as well as my grandmothers and grandfathers, all lived healthy lives until passing in their mid-to-late nineties. I couldn't recall any exceptions. *Why*, I asked?

I recognized that my entire family ate healthy Mediterranean diets and were physically active all day long. But the mechanism of it remained a mystery.

There must be something in the chemistry, I thought, *some molecule or grouping of molecules was responsible for creating a protective effect against the development of cardiovascular disease.*

Although I had no idea what this molecule might be, I believed that mammalian cells might be capable of producing it. I had not been in a position to pursue such a research project while in the drug industry, but in the academic setting, with the freedom to conduct whatever basic research one's heart desires, the sky was the limit.

During the first five years as an assistant and then associate professor, I established my research laboratory and learned the skills of teaching pharmacology to our second-year medical students. Though I'd long held the feeling that I wanted to teach, I did not realize how rewarding it could be until I did it. I never could have predicted how gratifying it would be to watch students nod and show expressions of satisfaction as I stood before the class of 150, attempting to explain principles of pharmacology and physiology. One of my favorite things was that every once in a while, during a silent moment while students were busy taking notes, I'd hear someone say to a classmate, "Oh, now I get it!"

By 1977, my basic research on cyclic GMP was flourishing, and I had published dozens of research articles in peer-reviewed scientific journals. But one thing was still lacking for me.

I wanted to teach the students all about cardiovascular drugs. After years of pestering, it finally happened. In 1978, the chairman of the department approached me and requested that I teach a portion of the lectures on cardiovascular drugs. He asked me which drugs in particular captured my interest. Since I had just started to study the vasodilator properties of nitroglycerin in my laboratory at precisely that time, I told him that I wanted to address vasodilator drugs and other drugs used to lower blood pressure. He approved and instructed me to prepare to deliver three or four lectures.

I spent a considerable amount of time in preparation, reviewing the entire scientific and medical literature on vasodilators and other drugs used clinically to lower the blood pressure in patients having high blood pressure or hypertension. One such drug was nitroglycerin.

I was surprised to see that the literature on nitroglycerin as a vasodilator was scant. I did read that the vasodilator properties of nitroglycerin were first recognized in Alfred Nobel's dynamite factories and found literature that explained that the physiology involving the action of nitroglycerin had been nicely worked out. For example, the anti-anginal effect of nitroglycerin was attributed to dilation of the veins instead of coronary arteries, as previously thought.

But we pharmacologists always want to understand the mechanism of action of drugs, and the vasodilators are no different. In teaching this subject, I spent ample time going over the mechanisms of drug action. However, when it came time to discuss nitroglycerin, there was no known molecular mechanism to explain to the students.

After my lecture on nitroglycerin, a student raised her hand and said, "Professor, you told us all about nitroglycerin and that it relieves angina by dilating the veins rather than the arteries. That's great stuff, but you didn't tell us *how* it relaxes vascular smooth muscle. What's the molecular mechanism by which nitroglycerin causes vasodilation?"

That was a great question that briefly caught me off guard. I told her and the class that the molecular mechanism of action of nitroglycerin was completely unknown. Many of the students questioned why absolutely nothing was known about a popular drug that had been prescribed for over a hundred years. Another student spoke out and insisted that ascertaining its mechanism of action couldn't be that difficult or too elusive for pharmacologists to unravel.

I was impressed by the directness of her comment, and, with that, I invited this student to work in my laboratory on a project to elucidate the mechanism of action of nitroglycerin. The class chuckled at my invitation, but I was sincere and would have gladly given her some of my laboratory space and guidance. She later refused my offer, stating that medical school was hard enough, and she did not believe that she could handle both her studies and laboratory research.

Later that afternoon, when I returned to my office, I was struck by the disappointment the students had expressed that I could not explain how nitroglycerin works as a vasodilator. Without delay, I embarked on a comprehensive literature search for anything I could find that might explain how nitroglycerin relaxes vascular smooth muscle. But I could find no adequate explanation. The mechanism of action of nitroglycerin was a total mystery. *Imagine the impact of not knowing,* I thought. *How many lives are being lost because we don't understand this?* And so, to relieve stress, I turned, once again, to Elton John so that I could get nitroglycerin out of my mind for a while.

Listening to "Don't Go Breaking My Heart" and "Sorry Seems to Be the Hardest Word," I made a permanent mental note of my concerns and hoped that the opportunity might arise in the future for my laboratory to figure out how this drug works.

Despite my close bond with Heather, Jan and I had become increasingly distant over the years since moving to New Orleans. Her concern that I was too focused on work and didn't pay enough attention to them became a point of contention that we couldn't seem to get past.

Exactly seven years into our marriage, we decided it was best to part ways. Heather was nearly five years old at this point and couldn't understand what was happening. Jan took primary custody of Heather, and though we worked out a compromise so that I could see Heather over the weekends, the pain of not having her around was almost too much to bear. My time with Heather soon became the highlight of my week, and I spent the rest of my time completely enveloped in my work.

The Research Begins

My first research project at Tulane Medical School in 1973 focused on cyclic GMP, and my collaboration with others at Tulane proved to be successful in revealing some of the signaling properties of cyclic GMP. However, after about four years, we still lacked any trace of evidence to support my long-standing theory about a unique molecule that could protect us against cardiovascular disease. But then, a candidate for such a molecule appeared in a research paper published in 1977, although I did not appreciate its significance at the time.

A chemical known as nitric oxide (NO) was demonstrated to activate an enzyme, guanylate cyclase, that catalyzes the formation of cyclic GMP in mammalian cells. This was an exciting finding because now we knew of a molecule, NO, that could increase cyclic GMP production in cells and thereby provide the opportunity to study the effects, if any, of increases in cyclic GMP levels on cell function. This is exactly the kind of chemical tool one needed to study the physiological relevance of cyclic GMP in tissues.

Adding NO to airway (trachea) smooth muscle was reported to increase tissue cyclic GMP, and this was accompanied by relaxation of the smooth muscle. The increase in cyclic GMP was severalfold, and the smooth muscle relaxation was profound, even with a low concentration of NO. I was struck with the observations that NO was an active and potent smooth muscle relaxant. This was the first pharmacological effect described for NO.

Still, I did not immediately conclude from these observations that NO might be the miracle molecule I was looking for. The reason was that nitric oxide, which is a gas just like oxygen, was well known to be a component of air pollution, where it reacts with the oxygen in the air to produce a different molecule, nitrogen dioxide (NO_2), also known as acid rain. Since NO_2 is such a deadly toxic gaseous molecule, no one in their right mind was thinking about the possibility that NO might have any biological significance. That is, it was inconceivable that NO could exist naturally in mammals. Nevertheless, something about the data captured my interest. I just couldn't put my finger on it.

Since my laboratory had been studying cyclic GMP for several years, these new observations with NO pointed us in a different direction, namely, smooth muscle relaxation. The published work involved studies on airway smooth muscle, but I wondered about vascular smooth muscle. Would arterial and venous smooth muscle also relax (widen or dilate) in response to added NO? Could NO be a vasodilator in addition to being a bronchodilator? If such turned out to be the case, this would mean that NO could both lower blood pressure and increase blood flow to various organs in the body. *This would be exciting pharmacology*, I thought, and I decided to explore this further.

Accordingly, I set up the necessary experiments to test this hypothesis. Working together with Professor Phil Kadowitz and Carl Gruetter, his postdoctoral fellow within the Department of Pharmacology, we went on to demonstrate that nitric oxide interacts with arterial and venous tissues to elevate intracellular levels of cyclic GMP and thereby bring about relaxation of the vascular smooth muscle.

At about this time, a report was published that nitroglycerin stimulates the production of cyclic GMP in blood vessels, which is associated with the relaxation of vascular smooth muscle. *Could this be*, I thought, *the long-awaited mechanism by which nitroglycerin causes vasodilation of the arteries and veins?* At this time, in 1978, I recalled that it had been about a hundred years prior that William Murrell, an English physician and clinical pharmacologist, discovered the vasodilator properties of nitroglycerin in the dynamite factories of Alfred Nobel. Coincidentally, this report on nitroglycerin appeared only a few weeks after I gave a lecture to the medical students at Tulane, during which I explained that the mechanism of vasodilator action of nitroglycerin was a mystery. Here was my timely opportunity to investigate and, perhaps, elucidate the mechanism of action of this drug.

In view of our successful early experiments on nitric oxide, and our hypothesis that nitroglycerin might work through a cyclic GMP mechanism, I wrote an NIH research grant proposal in an attempt to obtain funds to carry out this research. Most of the funding for biomedical research in the US was, and still is, provided by the various institutes within the NIH, on a competitive basis. Since my basic research program centered around the cardiovascular system, my funding came from the National Heart, Lung, and Blood Institute (NHLBI). My prior NIH grants dealing with cyclic GMP all had been approved and funded. However, this new grant application would deal with nitric oxide, a new field in biomedical research, and I was uncertain whether we'd get the funding.

Once an NIH grant application is submitted, it usually takes about five or six months to learn whether that grant has been approved and awarded. Notifications were sent out by mail in those days and printed on pink-colored paper, referred to as the "pink sheet." Some called them the dreaded pink sheet. One day, as I picked up my incoming mail in the departmental office, I recognized a government-printed envelope from the NIH. I knew exactly what would be inside. My anxiety level began to rise. I kept telling myself to relax because my cyclic GMP research had been productive, and my research proposal involving NO was logical and straightforward, at least to me.

I opened the envelope, took out the pink sheet, and started to read it. "What?" I said out loud. "This can't be!" I glanced at my score and saw that it was not high enough for funding. My heart sank, and I started to take long, deep breaths. This was the first time that any of my grant proposals was not approved and funded.

I went on to read the entire evaluation report and learned that the major concern of the reviewers was the apparent lack of physiological relevance of NO. They questioned why I should receive competitive government money to study a noxious gas found in the earth's atmosphere.

One of several disconcerting comments was: "The NHLBI is not in a position to fund biologically irrelevant science dealing with atmospheric gases."

Another was: "The PI (Principal Investigator, i.e., *me*) has apparently lost his ability to focus his research on biologically relevant pharmacology. He would be better off submitting this proposal to an agency interested in air pollution."

It was this second comment that drove me up the wall. But anger quickly turned to concern because I was uncertain of how I would be able to continue my work on nitric oxide.

I kept reading the pink sheet over and over again, trying to understand the reviewers' remarks. What the reviewers failed to understand, I thought, was that I was going to use NO only as a pharmacological tool to stimulate the production of cyclic GMP in various tissues of the cardiovascular system. My intent was to determine the actions, and therefore, the physiologic relevance of cyclic GMP. After thinking about this for a while, I thought perhaps I should have focused my proposal on cyclic GMP instead of NO.

The bottom line was that I would not have any funds to support my work on NO. Deep down, I knew that NO could be the key to developing a greater understanding of how the cardiovascular system is regulated in health and disease. Somehow, I needed to raise the funds to study NO. I had to figure out how I could accomplish this, and quickly!

Then I had an idea to use some funds from my other existing research grants. I did not feel this was unethical because my proposed work on NO was closely related to the cardiovascular work covered by my existing grants.

However, before engaging in these experiments, another stumbling block presented itself. A manuscript on nitric oxide that I had submitted for publication in a highly ranked scientific journal (*Nature*) had been rejected.

Similar to the language in the "pink sheet," the journal editor explained that "the editorial board believes nitric oxide is physiologically irrelevant and would not be of any interest to the average reader of the journal."

My face began to flush and not from embarrassment. *What do they want from me?* I thought. *Why is the scientific community so dead set against learning about the biological properties of NO?*

Once again, the reviewers failed to appreciate NO as a pharmacological. I felt that the reviewers of both my grant and manuscript had great difficulty getting past the tree branches in order to see the entire forest and what it had to offer.

I was determined to get my first paper on NO published, no matter which journal. Accordingly, I wrote up the manuscript for submission to a new and less well-known journal, and it was published. At least I got the work out there for any interested reader to study and draw their own conclusions.

I was determined not to allow any of this negativity to interfere with or interrupt my work. I firmly believed that studying NO, despite it being a noxious gas, was important in developing a better understanding of cell signaling in mammalian tissues. I'd never given up before, and I was not about to give up then.

PART III:
A Nobel Discovery

"Do not go where the path may lead, go instead where
there is no path and leave a trail."
— *Ralph Waldo Emerson*

Chapter 8:
My Basic Research on Nitric Oxide

T he early morning hours are when I do my most creative thinking, which is mandatory to conceive and design key experiments in the laboratory. One morning, while planning experiments involving cyclic GMP, I reread a report on nitroglycerin that had been published a few weeks prior. The data revealed that the addition of nitroglycerin to isolated blood vessels in an *in vitro* experimental setup causes smooth muscle relaxation associated with an elevation in cyclic GMP levels. It was already well known that nitroglycerin causes smooth muscle to relax, but what was new was that nitroglycerin caused a simultaneous increase in cyclic GMP levels in the smooth muscle. The obvious question: Could cyclic GMP be responsible for the vasodilator action of nitroglycerin?

Then it occurred to me that perhaps we should study the chemistry of nitroglycerin more closely to try to get insight as to how it could stimulate the production of cyclic GMP. I looked at the chemistry of nitroglycerin, of which I was familiar, and noted that this small molecule contained three nitrate ester (ONO_2) groups, as illustrated in Figure 1.

Suddenly, an idea came to mind. What if one or more of these ONO_2 groups is converted to NO? *This is a reasonable possibility,* I thought, *since the ONO_2 obviously contains NO built into the molecule.* Arguing that the ONO_2 might be converted to NO inside cells of the smooth muscle, it was easy to reason that the NO generated could then elevate cyclic GMP levels. In turn, the cyclic GMP would cause the arterial smooth muscle to relax. If this were the case, it would clearly explain the mechanism of vasodilator action of nitroglycerin.

We set up a biological experiment to determine whether the addition of nitroglycerin to isolated arteries could trigger the formation of nitric oxide in the arterial smooth muscle cells. Nitroglycerin was added to pieces of artery in a glass chamber under conditions simulating the biological environment. The tissues were then analyzed for nitric oxide and other possible metabolites of nitroglycerin that might be formed.

The results provided an exciting breakthrough in pharmacology. Nitroglycerin was metabolized in the arterial smooth muscle cells to NO. The NO produced in this reaction came from the nitroglycerin, as illustrated in Figure 1, and the accompanying product was the predicted metabolite of nitroglycerin.

$$
\begin{array}{ccc}
\text{H}_2\text{C-ONO}_2 & & \text{H}_2\text{C-OH} \\
| & & | \\
\text{HC-ONO}_2 & \longrightarrow & \text{HC-ONO}_2 \quad + \quad \boxed{\text{NO}} \\
| & & | \\
\text{H}_2\text{C-ONO}_2 & & \text{H}_2\text{C-ONO}_2
\end{array}
$$

FIGURE 1.
METABOLISM OF NITROGLYCERIN TO NO IN VASCULAR SMOOTH MUSCLE CELLS

Nitric oxide is relatively small when compared to other molecules in nature. For example, nitric oxide consists of only two atoms, one atom of nitrogen (N) and one atom of oxygen (O). The chemical abbreviation of nitric oxide is, therefore, NO.

The next question to answer was whether the nitric oxide formed from nitroglycerin is actually responsible for the vasodilator action of the nitroglycerin. The only way to know for sure was to purchase authentic NO gas and test it in the lab. And so, we did, and we found that NO, added to isolated segments of artery or vein, caused a complete relaxation of the smooth muscle. The other product of the reaction illustrated in Figure 1 was inactive in that it did not produce any effects on the vascular smooth muscle. The obvious conclusion from these experiments was that NO is the active component in nitroglycerin that causes vasodilation.

After a few more experiments to tie things together, I prepared a manuscript for submission to one of the most respected journals of pharmacology in the US, the *Journal of Pharmacology and Experimental Therapeutics*. This time, I truly believed that our work on NO would be published because we had elucidated the mechanism of vasodilator action of nitroglycerin by releasing NO as its active principle. This work was good solid pharmacology and solved a one-hundred-year mystery. This time, our manuscript was accepted and published. I had hoped that this publication would open the door to future publications on NO and perhaps also to NIH funding of projects involving NO. I felt relaxed and, finally, my anxiety began to dissipate.

Whenever I use the words nitric oxide, a great majority of people think I am referring to "nitrous oxide." I have to remind them that, while they may sound the same, nitric oxide and nitrous oxide are two completely different molecules. They are both gases, but that's where their similarity ends. Nitrous oxide, commonly referred to as "laughing gas," is a gaseous anesthetic agent that is commonly used by dentists and dental hygienists to provide patients with some pain relief during dental procedures. Nitrous oxide is also used as an inhalational anesthetic in the operating room in preparation for surgical patients to receive additional anesthetic agents prior to surgery. This anesthetic gas is highly stable in the presence of air or oxygen. That is, nitrous oxide does not decompose in the presence of oxygen. Unlike nitrous oxide, nitric oxide is highly unstable because it reacts rapidly with oxygen and is destroyed within seconds.

To ensure our study was correct, we conducted additional experiments in which we added nitric oxide to isolated arteries and veins, recorded smooth muscle relaxation responses, and measured tissue levels of cyclic GMP. The data obtained were clear. The addition of NO caused a prompt elevation of cyclic GMP levels, which immediately preceded the onset of smooth muscle relaxation. The story was now complete. Nitroglycerin relaxes arteries and veins by being converted in smooth muscle cells to NO, which then stimulates the production of cyclic GMP, which, in turn, causes smooth muscle relaxation.

The medical significance of this discovery is that, after one hundred years of using the drug clinically, the mechanism of vasodilator action of nitroglycerin was finally revealed. If only nitric oxide could be used as a drug, it might be more suitable than its parent molecule, nitroglycerin, as a drug for treating hypertension or other cardiovascular diseases. However, nitric oxide is an unstable gas and cannot, obviously, be administered orally or intravenously. And so, we still use nitroglycerin to this day.

When one takes a nitroglycerin tablet, the drug finds its way first into the bloodstream and then into the smooth muscle cells of the arteries and veins, where it is metabolized or converted to nitric oxide. This nitric oxide then rapidly elevates cyclic GMP levels and causes the arteries and veins to widen (vasodilation), thereby lowering the blood pressure and increasing blood flow. Moreover, these findings provided the motivation to study in depth other potential effects of nitric oxide, acting via cyclic GMP, on biological tissues, especially blood vessels.

But what intrigued me most about nitric oxide was its capacity to activate the enzyme *guanylate cyclase*. I wanted to focus my attention on the mechanisms involved. Nitric oxide markedly activates guanylate cyclase several hundredfold, thereby resulting in the production of relatively large quantities of cyclic GMP. Activating an enzyme is like adding much more enzyme to the mix, and this is how more product is formed in the reaction. This remarkable effect of NO has intrigued me since it was first reported by Professor Ferid Murad in 1977.

In designing my approach to experiments that would help to ascertain the precise mechanism by which nitric oxide could possibly activate an enzyme protein, we needed to purify guanylate cyclase to homogeneity (one single protein instead of a crude mixture of many proteins).

I started a collaborative effort with a professor of biochemistry at Tulane, Bill Baricos, and together, we developed several methods of enzyme protein purification. Nearly every step of the procedure had to be conducted in the cold room, where the temperature was maintained between 0°C to 4°C, which is 32°F to 39°F for five or six days and nights. In addition, I recruited one technician and one graduate student to work with my biochemist colleague and me, and the project was a go. Well, almost.

Before we got started, I realized that I was not certain about the best purification techniques to utilize. Although I had some expertise in purifying proteins, it was not extensive enough. Most importantly, I was unfamiliar with the column chromatography method for purifying proteins, which is what we needed to employ if we wanted to purify guanylate cyclase to homogeneity.

As I sat in my office, contemplating this potential roadblock, I suddenly realized that I might be able to get advice from someone nearby, in fact, right across the street. The Veterans Administration Hospital, which was also a research center, happened to be where Dr. Andrew Schally had several large laboratories focused on the purification of peptides by column chromatography. Dr. Schally was a renowned expert in this area of basic research.

He was well known for having enormous, seemingly endless, glass columns that he used to separate and purify peptides. Some of these chromatographic columns were twenty-five feet long and twelve inches in diameter and had to be set up using three laboratories, one floor on top of the other, by boring holes in the ceilings/floors to accommodate the oversized columns vertically. I was struck by his motivation to accomplish what he set out to do.

The following morning, I walked over to see Dr. Schally. I found him in one of his laboratories speaking with several people. Finishing his conversation, Schally started to walk out the door. Just before he reached the exit, he saw me, looked right at me, ignored me, and continued out the door.

I followed him out and asked if I might have a word with him about his column chromatography.

He stopped and turned around to face me.

I continued by telling him my name and that I was on the faculty at Tulane, right across the street, and proceeded to explain, "I am working on a research project that involves protein purification, and I wanted to ask you some questions about column chromatography, an area in which you are an expert."

"You are correct. I am the world's expert on column chromatography. I have the largest and most efficient chromatography columns."

I was taken aback. Schally appeared to be arrogant and not at all friendly, but I hoped he would be willing to help me out.

He continued, "What are you trying to purify? I don't purify proteins; only very small molecules like peptides."

I told him that the protein I was working with was guanylate cyclase, a relatively large protein.

"I'm not an expert in enzyme protein or large protein purification," he said. "I can't help you."

As I started to speak again, he ignored me again and walked back toward his office. I followed him and tried to keep pace; I knew I needed to reach him before he shut himself in his office.

"I know your work, Dr. Schally, and I understand very well that you purify peptides from the pituitary gland and hypothalamus in the brain. I'm looking for help to purify a large protein. Might you be willing to allow me to come to your lab to observe your people using column chromatographic methods?"

"But I told you that we don't purify proteins, only peptides. You won't find anyone in my laboratory who works with proteins."

"I fully understand that, Dr. Schally. With all due respect, all I want to do is observe your chromatographic columns and study how your people use them to purify peptides. By observing them, I just might be able to improve how we apply such methods to proteins."

He stopped walking. It was obvious to me that he was irritated. I held my breath.

"Okay," he said.

Yes! His one-word answer was all I needed to take the next steps. Although I felt most uncomfortable begging him for assistance, I knew it had to be done if I was going to learn column chromatography from the best source possible.

During the next few months, two of my lab techs and I visited Schally's laboratory on a regular basis to learn how to perform column chromatography and several other techniques that we could adapt to purifying proteins. I was convinced that his methods would prove successful. Within a few months, we learned a great deal about chromatographic procedures, especially column chromatography. On several of my visits to his lab, Schally recognized me and said hello. But that's all. He was not one for social chit-chat.

A few months later, in October of 1977, I was heading over to his lab one morning when I noticed a crowd of people and lots of news reporters just outside the building. I wondered what the fuss was about. As I reached the crowd, I asked one of the reporters what was going on. She told me that Dr. Schally had just received the news from Stockholm that he was awarded the Nobel Prize in Physiology or Medicine. Since I was wearing my white lab coat, the reporter asked me if I worked with Dr. Schally. I told her not exactly, but I often visited his lab.

I stood around for at least an hour to see if I could sneak in and congratulate him myself.

Once I was able to enter the building, I pushed myself in between two reporters and wound up standing right in front of Dr. Schally, and I congratulated him.

Much to my surprise, he looked right at me, smiled, extended his hand for a handshake, and said, "Thank you very much."

I returned to my office feeling good about two things. First, Andrew Schally was awarded the Nobel Prize, which he richly deserved. Second, he finally spoke to me, and with a smile to boot! That day boosted my motivation and determination to launch our difficult but necessary project, the purification of guanylate cyclase.

About four months after learning several special techniques in Andrew Schally's laboratory, we successfully purified guanylate cyclase to homogeneity.

Of all the basic research projects I've ever been involved with in my research career, this one was the most stimulating but, at the same time, the most challenging. The experience reinforced the importance of working with experts in specific areas to develop the methodological techniques required to answer critical questions in biology and physiology. More often than not, I'd had to rely on the knowledge provided by other scientists to attain my goals in my laboratory. I could not have purified guanylate cyclase without the assistance of Andrew Schally. Similarly, a few years back, I could not have developed a new anti-inflammatory drug without the help of Chris de Duve.

In the final step of a five-day effort, we noted that the concentrated homogeneous protein solution was red in color. This surprised me because the great majority of purified proteins in solution are clear, with no color. The red color reminded me of concentrated solutions of hemoglobin, which also are red. Hemoglobin is the oxygen-carrying protein in red blood cells, and it gives them their bright red color. The specific component or molecule of hemoglobin that causes its red color is termed heme. In addition to hemoglobin, other proteins contain heme, and these proteins are also red. Such heme-containing proteins have been called, simply, hemeproteins. Therefore, we reasoned that the red color of guanylate cyclase could have been attributed to the presence of heme. Accordingly, we conducted the appropriate analytical experiments to determine whether, in fact, heme was present. The experimental results were clear. Guanylate cyclase was indeed a hemeprotein.

Every protein that contains heme performs a specific function. For example, the heme in hemoglobin binds oxygen, which is obtained in the lungs and transports the oxygen in the circulating red blood cells to all tissues and organs in the body. But it was also known that the heme of hemoglobin can bind NO and carbon dioxide. And so, the obvious question arose as to the function of the heme molecule in guanylate cyclase. Did this heme group also bind NO? Was the heme involved in enzyme activation by NO?

To answer these questions, we had to purify a great deal more guanylate cyclase so that we would have sufficient quantities of enzyme protein to work with and analyze. This was a significant amount of work, but it paid off. Eventually, we found that the heme group in guanylate cyclase was required for enzyme activation by NO.

Next, we needed to answer the one question I'd asked throughout my childhood and every day since: *Why?* In this particular case, *Why was heme required?*

At this time, I was fortunate to have a new postdoctoral fellow join my laboratory. Michael Wolin, who had a chemistry background, had just graduated from the biochemistry program at Yale University with a PhD in enzymology and wanted to learn more about biology and pharmacology. We sat down, and I explained what I wanted us to do regarding guanylate cyclase and the requirement of heme for enzyme activation by NO. We thought about the basic research project for a couple of weeks and then planned our course of action.

We used the technique of spectrophotometry to help us. Spectrophotometry is a method based on the quantitative analysis of molecules depending on how much light is absorbed by the molecule. An important physical-chemical principle in nature is that all compounds with a color absorb light, and the extent of absorption can be determined experimentally. Spectrophotometers measure the intensity of a light beam as a function of its color (wavelength of light). Tiny differences in color can be detected, recorded, and quantified by spectrophotometry.

In view of prior studies by others that NO could bind to the heme groups in hemoglobin, we set out to determine whether NO could also bind to the heme group in guanylate cyclase. After several experiments involving spectral analysis, we determined that NO binds to the iron atom located in the center of the heme molecule. This modified heme molecule is termed NO-heme. The overall conclusion we reached through our spectral experiments was that NO activates guanylate cyclase by heme-dependent mechanisms involving the binding of NO to heme iron.

During the subsequent two years, we were able to elucidate the precise molecular mechanism by which formation of NO-heme results in the activation of guanylate cyclase, thereby stimulating the production of cyclic GMP in cells. It was clear from our studies that the biological receptor for NO in guanylate cyclase was heme iron.

This would turn out to be a critically important discovery.

Chapter 9:
Connecting the Dots

The purification and characterization of guanylate cyclase, described earlier, took about three years. We initiated the project in late 1978 and obtained our first sample of purified enzyme in 1981. This particular project took most of our manpower and time, but it was well worth the effort.

Early in 1982, the chairman of the Department of Pharmacology informed me that we would have a special guest come by to visit the department later in April, a Professor John Vane who, at the time, was director of research at the Wellcome Foundation, located just outside of London. He was coming to New Orleans to attend an international conference and told our chairman that he wished to stop by to meet with some of the faculty at Tulane Medical Center.

I'd followed the work of John Vane since I was in graduate school in the 1960s. He was what I would term a classical pharmacologist, who used isolated organs and tissues under controlled conditions to study the impact of drugs and other chemicals on organ function. Although I was keen on using chemical approaches and had avoided isolated organ experiments, I admired and respected Dr. Vane for his pursuits—to raise and answer critically important questions in biology and physiology.

A great example: Vane assembled a team of pharmacologists, physiologists, and chemists to isolate, separate, purify, and synthesize the naturally occurring prostaglandins known at the time. The prostaglandins are a group of lipid molecules, some of which are produced at sites of inflammation, but nothing much was known about them at the time. Vane studied their pharmacology in a systematic manner and found that some of the prostaglandins provoked local inflammation, pain, and fever. He realized, as did many other pharmacologists, that aspirin is used as a drug for three major benefits—as an anti-inflammatory for treating arthritis and related inflammatory disease, an excellent analgesic for relieving all kinds of pain, and an antipyretic to lower body temperature during fever.

So, there we have it, as Vane would later say at many scientific conferences. Prostaglandins cause inflammation, pain, and fever, whereas aspirin prevents all three. Coincidence? No, not a chance.

Vane went on to consider a simple and logical question: Could aspirin be working therapeutically by inhibiting the production of prostaglandins? He tested his hypothesis, and the rest is history. Aspirin inhibits the production of prostaglandins in the body and thereby reduces or eliminates inflammation, pain, and fever. After a hundred years of the widespread use of aspirin, Vane was the one who finally elucidated the mechanism of action of aspirin.

I was hoping that I would have the opportunity to meet and chat with Professor Vane during his brief visit. This would be a good occasion to tell him about my work on nitric oxide and cyclic GMP and ask for his insight. Although I wasn't sure how much he knew about nitric oxide, I specifically wanted to share with him that nitric oxide is a vasodilator and that it also interferes with platelet function and, therefore, inhibits blood clotting. We also had discovered that nitric oxide increases cyclic GMP in platelets and is the molecule that creates these effects. I believed this would be of particular interest to Vane because of his studies with aspirin, which had been well known to inhibit platelet aggregation and local blood clotting. This is why aspirin was, and still is, used to prevent a second heart attack in patients with cardiac problems.

When Professor Vane came to my office, we exchanged greetings, and I kicked off the conversation by telling him how much I respected his work on the mechanism of action of aspirin, and then I asked, "What led you to decide to study the pharmacology of the prostaglandins in the first place?"

He wiggled around in his chair to get more comfortable. He paused for a few seconds, raised his arms to place his hands on the front edge of my desk, and answered, "Prostaglandins were first discovered in 1935 by Ulf von Euler, a Swedish pharmacologist, who I am certain you are aware of. At the time, prostaglandins were recognized to be lipid substances that occurred naturally in mammals, including humans. But no one knew much about their pharmacology except that they might function as hormones.

And so, I decided to begin studying their pharmacology in the mid-1960s."

"And when did you figure out that aspirin might work by inhibiting the production of these prostaglandins?"

Vane wiggled around in his chair once again and looked right at me. Then he rolled his eyes up, looking at the ceiling, as if trying to recall the exact date.

"1971," he said, and added, "During the subsequent few years, we elucidated the enzymatic machinery for prostaglandin synthesis and that aspirin inhibits the enzyme responsible for prostaglandin formation."

"Incredible!" I said as I shook my head. "It's astounding to me that it took nearly one hundred years to figure this out."

Then, I could no longer control my urge to ask, "Isn't that Nobel Prize material?"

He paused for a long moment, and then a grin broke through his normally serious visage, "*I* think so!" he said. "We'll just have to wait and see what happens."

"Professor Vane, your discoveries clearly demonstrated that the inhibition of prostaglandin formation results in the relief of inflammation, pain, and fever. This is what aspirin does, as you showed. I hope that the drug industry will take advantage of your discoveries by screening many compounds for their activity as inhibitors of prostaglandin formation. Such screening could reveal agents that might be much more potent and safer than aspirin."

It turns out that such screening procedures quickly led to the development of ibuprofen and naproxen as analgesic/anti-inflammatory drugs.

He then turned the tables. "What about your work, Dr. Ignarro?"

I immediately asked him to call me Lou. Then I explained nitric oxide and cyclic GMP and their biochemistry.

Shortly into my lecture, he interrupted me and said, "Lou, I know all that. What I want to know is *why* you are studying NO. Why NO, of all things? NO is a pollutant gas in our environment and does not exist naturally in cells, to the best of my knowledge. So, why are you studying it?"

His comments were loud, forceful, and almost brash. Indeed, his pronounced British accent made me feel like I was being deposed. But then I realized with a pleasantly surprised touch of pride that he must have been reading about my basic research.

"I am studying nitric oxide because I am impressed with its potency. Just vanishingly small amounts of NO dilate arteries and inhibit platelet function. I believe it possible that some molecule chemically related to NO, or which may be converted to NO, *might* exist in cells."

Vane nodded, and I continued, "I am a pharmacologist and, as such, I'm studying the pharmacology of NO. For example, what else does NO do in the body? NO inhibits platelet function, just like aspirin does. I want to determine whether such decreased platelet function results in the inhibition of blood clotting. After all, aspirin inhibits blood clotting by interfering with platelet function." I could tell by his expression that he was becoming more interested in what I had to say, but then I detected an abrupt about-face.

"Well. Tell me, Lou," Vane said. "Does NO exist naturally in mammalian cells?"

"No one has demonstrated this to date," I said, "but I want to pursue this possibility."

Vane nodded and said, "That might be an excellent idea, after all." Then he raised his voice again, and added, "So, why haven't you done this as yet?"

For a moment, I felt scolded for not having yet looked for NO in mammalian cells.

"The chemical properties of NO suggest that it might not be able to exist in cells because it is too unstable. This is why I've hesitated looking for NO in cells."

"It can't be *that* unstable," Vane argued. "When you add it to cells and tissues, it produces a pronounced pharmacologic effect, doesn't it?" His answer started to boost my confidence.

Vane then went on and posed that the widespread pharmacologic effects of NO make it worthwhile to perform experiments to determine whether NO can exist in cells.

"You are a pharmacologist, Lou. You must do this. That's what pharmacologists do."

I agreed. Moreover, I was pleased that he was starting to believe that NO was important to study.

He wished me the best of luck, and we shook hands. I thanked him for his visit, and as we started to walk out of my office,

I paused, turned to him, and said, "Professor Vane. One more comment, please. We have one thing in common. It took nearly a hundred years to reveal the mechanism of action of aspirin, which you accomplished. It also took nearly a hundred years to reveal the mechanism of action of nitroglycerin, which I accomplished."

He smiled at that and shook my hand again.

The visit by John Vane was highly motivating, especially because of the question he had posed to me: *Does nitric oxide exist naturally in mammalian cells?*

John Vane was awarded the Nobel Prize in Physiology or Medicine in 1982, just six months after his visit to Tulane. Soon after that, he was knighted by the Queen of England, and conferred the title of Sir.

I kept thinking about John Vane's strong recommendation that I pursue my belief that nitric oxide is produced by mammalian cells to regulate cardiovascular function. The problem was that I did not have the resources at Tulane to attack this problem head-on. Yes, I was pleased with the progress I'd made, but Vane's comments kept haunting me.

My experience in pharmacology taught me that whenever our cells respond to tiny amounts of a molecule, such as NO, it means that such a molecule is present naturally in our bodies and that we have receptors to bind to such molecules. I kept thinking,

We certainly have the receptors to bind to NO. Therefore, our blood vessels must produce nitric oxide.

But no one had ever demonstrated this before. Indeed, I had never heard anyone even talk about this. There was only one way to find out. I had to design experiments to determine whether arteries and veins could produce NO naturally. This was no easy task. After many months of thinking and planning, I realized that I had gone as far as I could in reasoning that NO might be produced in mammalian cells. The next step was to demonstrate this experimentally. I did not have the resources necessary at Tulane University to launch such a project, and this caused great frustration. Perhaps I needed to move to a different research center with more resources in order to test my hypothesis.

Dr. Robert Furchgott, who was professor of pharmacology at Brooklyn Downstate Medical Center in New York, had made a discovery two years earlier that the mechanism by which a neurotransmitter termed acetylcholine causes vasodilation of arteries. Although it had been known for over a hundred years that acetylcholine was a vasodilator (it caused vascular smooth muscle relaxation), no one had a clue about its mechanism of action or what caused it to do so. For example, when acetylcholine is injected intravenously in animals, it causes a profound vasodilation and consequent drop in blood pressure. On the other hand, when acetylcholine was tested *in vitro* by adding it to isolated strips or rings of artery, scientists observed no effect. No one had ever reported a relaxation response *in vitro*, as one would routinely see *in vivo* (in the living animal).

Furchgott demonstrated that, unlike many other vasodilators, acetylcholine required the presence of the endothelial cell layer in order to cause relaxation. This was the first demonstration that endothelial cells must be present and functional for acetylcholine to cause vascular smooth muscle relaxation. The schematic illustration in Figure 2 shows the location of the endothelial and smooth muscle cells in a typical segment of artery.

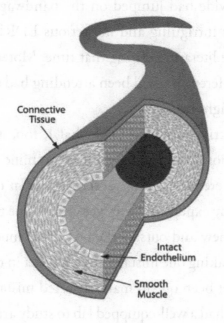

Connective
Tissue

Intact
Endothelium

Smooth
Muscle

FIGURE 2

In a series of classical pharmacological experiments, Dr. Furchgott and his colleagues demonstrated that acetylcholine first interacted with the endothelial cells to generate a factor or substance, which led to relaxation of the underlying smooth muscle cells. Not knowing the chemical nature of this factor, Furchgott named it endothelium-derived relaxing factor or EDRF.

In a subsequent series of elegant experiments, he showed that EDRF was a highly unstable substance. Once the EDRF was formed, this molecule lost all of its activity within a few seconds. Such chemical properties made it difficult, if not impossible, to isolate and identify or characterize. Within a year, dozens of laboratories worldwide had jumped on the bandwagon to attempt to identify this intriguing and mysterious EDRF, but nothing appeared in the literature during that time. Moreover, no one at the various conferences I had been attending had any concept of what EDRF might be.

I was so intrigued with EDRF that I, too, jumped in and made the decision to start a project to determine the identity of EDRF. But where was I going to start? In what direction was I going to take my experiments? It was clear to me that I'd have to do something new and outside the box. How much time would be wasted by making one mistake after another in trying to get on track? I've never been one to make repeated mistakes in the lab.

We already had a well-equipped lab to study arteries and veins *in vitro*, and the relaxant effects of nitric oxide. We began the project by trying to reproduce Furchgott's findings. After about six months of work, we were satisfied with our progress and felt confident that we could continue to study the production and actions of EDRF. By the fall of 1983, we had become proficient at studying vascular smooth muscle relaxation and other functions of arteries and veins, yet my frustration was beginning to mount because we still did not understand the nature of EDRF. Accordingly, I took a two-day vacation from my lab and spent many quiet hours at Audubon Park in New Orleans, where I gave serious thought to coming up with a definitive series of experiments that we could conduct to unravel the mysteries of EDRF.

I often find that a quiet outdoor environment is the best setting for critical thinking. The sounds of the trees blowing in the wind and the birds chirping provided me a relaxed state of mind that I found conducive to creative thinking. Like any scientist working in a specialized area where a significant discovery could be made, I wanted to be the first to identify the elusive EDRF. At this point, I recalled a famous saying from Winston Churchill that I modified slightly to be more fitting of a scientist: "The definition of a successful scientist is the ability to move from failure to failure without any loss of enthusiasm." I was determined to isolate and identify EDRF no matter what obstacles lay in front of me.

In addition to the soothing environment at Audubon Park, the music of Elton John inspired me to think clearly and plan incisive experiments. One of my favorite songs was "I'm Still Standing," released in 1983. This song was popular during one of the most challenging periods of my basic research career, where I had some ideas of what regulated cardiovascular function, but I was frustrated because I did not have all of the resources I needed to prove my theory. During times like this, I would play "I'm Still Standing" over and over again, and that helped me to cope.

One morning, while listening to Elton John's greatest hits, I conceived of a series of critical experiments that I believe needed to be performed. Shortly after, I went into the laboratory to meet with some of my people and asked them to perform these experiments.

In our first experiment, the objective was to try to reproduce Furchgott's original observations. We were successful, and Figure 3 illustrates the results of this experiment—that acetylcholine (in the bloodstream) binds to a membrane receptor (R), which then triggers the formation of EDRF in the endothelium. EDRF subsequently causes vascular smooth muscle relaxation. The mechanism by which EDRF caused relaxation was unknown (?). This was essentially the experiment that Robert Furchgott performed and published in 1980, and we were able to reproduce the results.

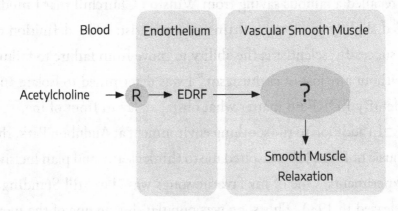

FIGURE 3

The next experiment we performed was to determine whether cyclic GMP might be involved in the relaxation process initiated by acetylcholine and EDRF. We were already experts in cyclic GMP research and had studied and published articles showing that NO causes vascular smooth muscle relaxation by mechanisms involving cyclic GMP formation. Since we knew that cyclic GMP is an intracellular signaling molecule that relaxes smooth muscle, we were curious if cyclic GMP might also be involved in the relaxation elicited by EDRF.

Figure 4 illustrates that acetylcholine, and presumably EDRF, caused an increase in the levels of cyclic GMP in the smooth muscle of the arterial rings, and this was directly associated with relaxation. As with the smooth muscle relaxation, the increase in cyclic GMP produced by acetylcholine was endothelium-dependent. But the question remained as to whether the increase in cyclic GMP was actually required for relaxation. In other words, was the cyclic GMP responsible for the relaxation effect of EDRF, or was the cyclic GMP doing something else at the same time?

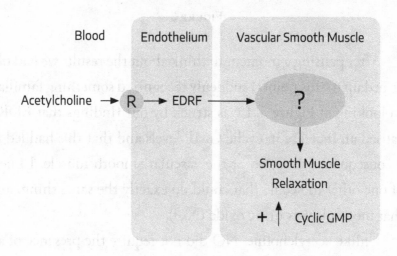

FIGURE 4

We performed additional experiments to determine whether cyclic GMP was required for the smooth muscle relaxation caused by acetylcholine. We found this to be the case, and Figure 5 illustrates that EDRF first promotes an increase in cyclic GMP levels, which then results in vascular smooth muscle relaxation. Meaning, the rise in cyclic GMP, triggered by EDRF, was required and responsible for the relaxation.

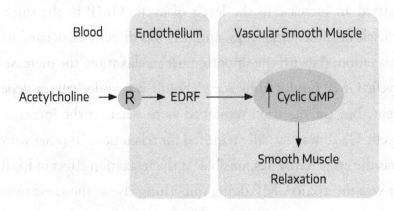

FIGURE 5

After pausing a moment to think about the results we had obtained up to this point, I suddenly recognized something familiar. In looking at Figure 5, I was struck by our findings that EDRF caused an increase in cyclic GMP levels and that this had led to a consequent relaxation of the vascular smooth muscle. I knew of one other molecule that could do exactly the same thing, and that molecule was nitric oxide (NO).

Unlike acetylcholine, NO did not require the presence of an intact functioning endothelium to increase cyclic GMP or cause smooth muscle relaxation. That is, NO caused endothelium-independent vascular smooth muscle relaxation. NO is a tiny molecule that can penetrate or permeate cell membrane barriers. This is illustrated in Figure 6, which shows that NO diffuses through cell membranes until it reaches and stimulates its target receptor, guanylate cyclase. The result is increased production of cyclic GMP. Clearly, the chemical behavior or properties of NO were very similar to those of EDRF (see Figure 5). Like NO, EDRF appeared to be a small diffusible molecule that moved from the endothelial cells into the underlying smooth muscle cells.

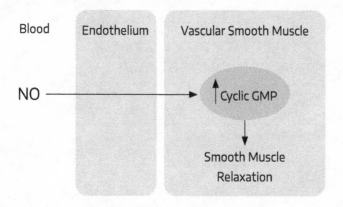

FIGURE 6

These experiments were tedious and time-consuming, but they yielded interesting and important information. We had elucidated the mechanism by which acetylcholine relaxes vascular smooth muscle and accounts for vasodilation in the mammalian species, thereby ending a hundred-year void in our understanding of how acetylcholine lowers blood pressure. Although this accomplishment was gratifying, it was incomplete. Our experiments still had failed to accomplish the original mission of these long and tiring studies, namely, to determine the chemical identity of EDRF. My frustrations continued to mount.

Chapter 10:
The Discovery that Led to the Nobel Prize

What in the world could EDRF be? I pored over our data and schematic illustrations again and again. First, I thought about EDRF, and then I thought about NO. I kept comparing the chemical properties of NO. Then I would look at the chemical properties of EDRF. I paced up and down the hallways and climbed up and down several flights of stairs to get my adrenaline flowing, and this helped my brain think more clearly, which made me more and more nervous. I went out into the stairwell for a few moments to pull myself together and regain my composure.

And then, it hit me.

The date was unforgettable. It was the early morning of May 31, 1984, my forty-third birthday. A few of the guys from the lab had organized a small birthday luncheon for me at a local Mexican restaurant near the university. But before I could leave for lunch, I needed to be alone and consolidate my thoughts about the chemical nature of EDRF.

Audubon Park was a great place to get in some early morning productive thinking. I grabbed a legal pad and a pencil and divided the page into two columns. The left-hand column, I labeled EDRF, and at the top of the right-hand column, I wrote NO.

I first listed each of the properties of EDRF that we had learned from our experiments. My plan for the right-hand column was to make a check mark next to the properties of EDRF that matched those of NO, and to write an X if there was no match. When I was done, all the marks in the NO column were check marks.

"Oh my God," I said. "Oh my God!" I kept saying out loud. "Oh my God! That's it, that's it! EDRF is NO! EDRF is NO!" All along, EDRF and NO were one and the same. What took us so damn long to recognize this?

A rough account of my thoughts, as I recall them, is presented in the table.

Clearly, the pharmacological, physiological, and biochemical evidence all pointed to the identical nature of EDRF and nitric oxide. The two were indistinguishable. However, such evidence was not enough to state unequivocally that EDRF was the same as NO. I had to make a positive "chemical" identification of EDRF as NO.

Knowing that this would take time, my anxiety level was once again on the rise because I knew that we could not publish that EDRF is the same chemical molecule as NO until we had performed the definitive chemical experiments. By this time, it was close to noon, and I headed to my birthday lunch at Pancho's.

Lou Ignarro
May 31, 1984
Comparison of EDRF vs. NO

EDRF	**NO**
1. Chemically unstable	✓
2. Half-life = 3 - 5 seconds	✓
3. Reducing agents (DTT, ascorbate) increase stability	✓
4. Oxidizing agents (O_2^{-}, manganese) decrease stability	✓
5. Readily diffuses through biologic membranes	✓
6. Activates cytosolic guanylate cyclase	✓
7. Stimulates intracellular cyclic GMP production	✓
8. Chemically reacts with iron and sulfur species	✓
9. Readily oxidized to nitrite (NO_2^{-}) and nitrate (NO_3^{-})	✓
10. Relaxes vascular smooth muscle	✓

CONCLUSIONS: EDRF appears to be NO. Next experiment must be to chemically identify EDRF as NO.

During our tasty lunch, my people sensed that something important was on my mind. They also noted that I'd broken from the norm and told everyone to order an alcoholic drink at lunch. We enjoyed a few sips of our drinks before I started talking about the exciting data that we had amassed during the past few months.

I began by reminding everyone of the unstable chemical properties of both NO and EDRF and went on to recap our observations that EDRF, like NO, causes an increase in cyclic GMP followed by vascular smooth muscle relaxation. As I was about to continue, the light bulbs must have started to go off, because one person at the table interrupted by stating that the properties of EDRF are the same as those for NO. The others agreed. I then asked the question: "Well then, do you believe that EDRF is NO?"

Everyone agreed and started applauding. The applause was followed by the group regaling me with the "Happy Birthday" song.

"But we're not there yet," I said and followed up by asking if anyone could see any differences in properties between EDRF and NO, or if anyone could tell me why EDRF might not be NO. Everyone agreed that the experimental evidence strongly suggested that EDRF was NO. I told the group that we needed to devise chemical experiments to prove the identity of EDRF, and quickly.

The Search for Proof

While I was working on the techniques that we needed to perform the next series of experiments, I was also writing up a research paper for publication of the experiments and data obtained thus far. However, it occurred to me that I would not be able to conclude or even suggest that EDRF is NO because of the lack of definitive chemical evidence. My fear was that the knowledgeable reader might look at our data and conclude, just as I did, that EDRF must be NO. That reader might then quickly perform and publish some definitive chemical experiments and beat us to the punch. I did not know what to do, and so I decided to take a week off to plan how we were going to make a chemical identification of EDRF.

My strategy was to use two different methods that were capable of detecting and quantifying small amounts of NO. One method was spectrophotometry, which detects specific substances based on the absorption of light by the sample being tested. The other method was chemiluminescense detection, which detects light emitted by the sample undergoing a chemical reaction. Both methods can be highly selective for detecting and measuring nitric oxide. The caveat was that I had neither the necessary expertise to use these methods, nor did I know of anyone else at Tulane University who could do it. It became utterly clear that I had to relocate to a much larger university with more advanced departments that I could interact with.

I vividly recalled when Sir John Vane had spoken with me and strongly recommended that I pursue my vision that nitric oxide is produced by mammalian cells. My thought was to telephone Professor Vane and run my idea by him that EDRF might be NO. It would be reassuring if he thought my reasoning was sound. Though I was afraid of sharing this potentially groundbreaking hypothesis with anyone outside my lab, I reasoned that he was an esteemed Nobel Laureate and likely to keep a secret. And so, I called him in London. Luckily, he was in his office.

"Lou. It's very nice to hear from you. To what do I owe this call?"

"Hello, Sir John," I said, to which he immediately told me to address him as John.

"Congratulations on the Nobel Prize, John. I'm sure that you've been busier than ever during the past two years, so I won't keep you long," I said. "The other reason I'm calling is to run an idea by you if you have time. I promise to be brief."

"Certainly! Do continue."

"I have good reason to believe that NO does, in fact, exist naturally in mammalian cells."

"Go on ..." he said. I briefly told him that we'd studied and compared the actions of EDRF and NO and found them to be virtually identical, both pharmacologically and chemically. And then I got to the main point of my call. "John, I believe, on the basis of my experiments, that EDRF is NO. All along, NO has been masquerading as EDRF. I wanted your opinion of my hypothesis."

"I believe that you could be correct. I've been following the EDRF field and, now that you mention it, EDRF behaves a lot like nitric oxide. Lou, if I were you, I'd get on this right away," he said with some urgency. "Even without seeing your data, you've convinced me that your idea could likely be correct. Let me know if I can help you in any way."

I thanked him for the reassuring discussion, and we hung up. I noticed I was sweating profusely. I had absolutely no doubt that I had to relocate my laboratory to a larger, more technologically advanced university to accomplish my goal. And I needed to do it soon. But where would I go?

Chapter 11:
Confirmation

T he University of California, Los Angeles (UCLA) had become a favorite spot for me to go to when I'd visit my mom, dad, and brother, who all had relocated to LA at about the time I went to New Orleans, in 1973. On occasion, I would drive over to the university and visit with friends and colleagues. I had been impressed with the incredible resources available to researchers, as well as their vast expertise in areas so important to my own research such as physiology, biochemistry, chemistry, and immunology.

In the spring of 1984, I received terrible news. My dad was gravely ill and would likely pass away within a few days. I made immediate arrangements to fly to Los Angeles to see him, but he passed two days before I arrived. It had been more than six months since I last visited my parents, and I did not get to see him one last time.

Attending and participating in my dad's wake and funeral were very difficult for me. Mom could see that I was falling apart, and she held my arm as we approached Dad in an open casket in the front of the visitation room. On seeing his face, I wept openly in the room sitting about sixty relatives and friends. I had known this day would eventually come, but I did not know how I would handle it.

In the gathering that followed, I managed to hold myself together and explain to everyone what a kind, understanding, and loving father I had. My memories were vivid of how many times he got me out of trouble with Mom over my explosive chemistry experiments. I explained to some of my relatives how he always supported me in anything I set out to do: how he built me a wooden rocket so I could test out the rocket fuel I had manage to make and how he forgave me for demolishing the backyard fireplace-bar-b-que with a large firecracker, or small bomb, that I had made.

During the funeral mass that followed, I could not stop thinking about how much my dad supported me in any science experiment I performed. I remembered when he assisted me in the outdoor experiment that I had planned to test my hypothesis that light traveled faster than sound. He had no idea what we were doing. But after I explained the experimental results to him, he said to me, "Oh, now I understand." Just the thought of his voice started the tears flowing again.

In contrast, I could not grasp that Dad was no longer here with us. But knowing that he was such a good man, I also knew that he was now in a better place.

Between the guilt I felt in not being closer to my dad before his untimely passing and the respect I had for UCLA's science department, I knew UCLA was the place for me. Unfortunately, there were no open faculty positions in the Department of Pharmacology. Then, I had an idea.

During my postdoctoral fellowship at the NIH, I had met and befriended another chemical pharmacologist who was planning to engage in an academic career at UCLA. During our time serving as committee members together, Professor Art Cho had shared with me how much he enjoyed working at UCLA for many reasons, including the vast resources and teaching opportunities. I planned on approaching Art to see whether the Department of Pharmacology would consider creating a faculty position and recommending me for an appointment as professor.

I told Art that I would like to give a seminar lecture during one of my visits to Los Angeles, and the department would not be obligated to pay me a dime. He agreed, and I visited UCLA in the late summer of 1984, just months after Dad's passing.

I devoted a great deal of time and effort in preparing what I hoped would turn out to be a pivotal talk. It would have to be exciting and novel if I were to impress the audience, especially the Department of Pharmacology and its chairman, Professor Donald Jenden. I focused my talk on the important discoveries I had made to date. I needed to convince the audience that

I was uniquely qualified to continue to make pivotal discoveries in pharmacology and physiology.

In my talk, I addressed our discovery of the pharmacological mechanism of action of nitroglycerin, namely, that nitroglycerin is metabolized to NO. I also explained our discoveries that NO causes an increase in cyclic GMP levels, which then results in vasodilation and inhibition of platelet function.

It was one of the best talks I had ever given. The audience clearly was excited by my presentation. This enabled me to relax a bit, but the next important step was yet to come.

Following my talk, I met with Art Cho and Professor Don Jenden. Twenty minutes into our relaxed discussion about many different matters, I inquired whether there was a faculty position available in the department. I saw that I'd caught them by surprise.

"Why do you ask?" Professor Jenden said. "Are you interested?"

I said I was indeed interested and went on to explain that Tulane University did not have the resources I needed to extend and expand my basic research projects. I did not reveal my hypothesis that EDRF might be nitric oxide.

Professor Jenden indicated that there were no faculty positions currently open but that he could talk with the dean of the School of Medicine about the possibility of granting another faculty position to the department. If the dean, Professor Sherman Mellinkoff, was inclined to agree, then I would still have to formally apply, together with other potential candidates who might be interested in the same faculty position.

After spending most of the afternoon chatting with other faculty in the department, I was called into the chairman's office and given the good news that Dean Mellinkoff had agreed to give the department one more slot for a newly appointed faculty member. They asked me to submit a formal application to be considered. About three months later, I was invited back to UCLA to give another lecture and meet with the members of the search committee.

My interview with the Pharmacology Search Committee was scheduled to occur immediately after my lecture, which they all would attend. Considering that this upcoming lecture might make the difference as to whether I'd be accepted to UCLA or not, I gave a lot of consideration to what I would talk about. I made a point not to reveal my idea that EDRF was NO, as I did not have the evidence to support such a claim. My talk was followed by a very active Q&A with the search committee's five members. Three of the five were experts in vascular physiology, and the remaining two were biochemists. They all fired questions at me for about an hour, and I relished the interaction.

All of their questions were right on the mark, but one question really caught my attention. Despite my avoiding any comparison of EDRF to NO throughout my lecture, one committee member asked me if I had any evidence that NO might exist in cells. I told him no, but that I wanted to focus my future experiments on that very topic. Continuing, I indicated that the major reason for my desire to move my research lab to UCLA was that I believed I could answer that pivotal question here, on the UCLA campus. Another committee member asked me why I felt that UCLA was so special in completing this project. I told the group that the departments of chemistry and biochemistry at UCLA were superb and had all the resources I would need to get the job done. I believe that my response scored lots of points.

Once I returned to New Orleans, I waited. Eight weeks seemed like eight years. I could not eat or sleep well because all I had in my mind was getting out of town and beginning a new life in California. Moreover, my anxiety was compounded by the necessity that I not share this pending decision with anyone at Tulane.

Leaving New Orleans also meant leaving my daughter. One day, I picked her up and took her to the park, where I explained that I might be leaving New Orleans and moving to Los Angeles. I wasn't sure how she would react, but much to my relief, her response was, "I can't wait to visit you in LA!"

The Long-Awaited Envelope

Finally, the news came in the form of a letter from the chairman of the Department of Pharmacology at UCLA. After fidgeting with the envelope for twenty minutes like a nervous junior in high school receiving a letter from their top-choice college, I finally opened it and read the contents. Though several qualified candidates had applied, they had selected me! I was ecstatic over the decision, and my anxiety dissipated, but not for long.

Although I was excited about moving to California, I was not happy about having to face the chairman of the Department of Pharmacology, as well as everyone in my laboratory, to inform them of my decision to leave Tulane. I felt great consternation wondering whom I should inform first: Chairman Jim Fisher or the people in my lab? I decided to settle with my chairman first. What would I tell him? What was a good reason for me to resign from Tulane University? He'd always treated me fairly and with great respect. *Well,* I thought, *just tell him the truth. After all, it's not because of Jim that I'm leaving Tulane.*

After getting my thoughts together, I started walking to the chairman's office. I hesitated before entering his office, but I quickly regrouped, took a deep breath, and walked through the open door. "Jim," I said. "Do you have a few moments, please? I need to tell you something important."

Jim smiled and said, "Of course, Lou! I have all afternoon for you, if you need it."

My God, I thought. *This had better not take all afternoon!*

"Jim, after many months of thought, I have decided to leave New Orleans and move to Los Angeles." I paused for a moment because it was clear that Jim was in a state of shock.

"What?" he said. "Why would you want to do that? Your academic career here at Tulane has blossomed. You have become internationally recognized for your research, and here at Tulane, you are one of the very best teachers in the medical school. Why Los Angeles?"

"I have accepted a position as a professor of pharmacology at the UCLA School of Medicine, and I'll be leaving in about three months."

He asked me if I was going as chairman of the department, and I said no, just as a professor.

"But that's merely a lateral move. Why would you do that?"

"No," I said. "It's not a lateral move. I am going to UCLA because I need certain resources for my research that Tulane cannot provide, such as strong departments of chemistry and physiology. Here at Tulane, pharmacology is one of the top departments in the country, thanks to you, but the other departments are quite weak. You see, Jim, I am at a critical stage in my research where I absolutely must collaborate closely with top chemists and physiologists in order to unravel the mysteries of NO."

After a long pause, Jim said that he understood but was disappointed to lose me. He walked me to the hallway outside his office and wished me the best of luck.

"Whew," I said under my breath as I started to walk away. I did what had to be done, and it worked out okay. But next, I had to tell my people, and that was not going to be any easier. I felt that my graduate students would be fine because they were finishing up their PhD dissertation research and already writing their final dissertations. My lab technicians were excellent, and I was confident that I could get other labs in the medical school to hire them. I was not worried about anyone, but I was still anxious about having to inform them.

I walked into one of my labs and found everyone present. Without delay, I asked them to gather around me, and I told them about my plans. A long pause followed, and there were lots of questions of concern, together with some tears. But over the next two hours, I managed to calm everyone and explain why everything would work out just fine. It took a couple of weeks for me to find alternate positions for my lab personnel. Each of my people was superb in the lab, and all the faculty in the medical school knew that.

UCLA

On May 15, 1985, I started my new academic position as professor of pharmacology at the UCLA School of Medicine. Two weeks earlier, I had driven all the way from New Orleans to LA with my daughter, who was excited to help me move into a new condominium I had purchased in Encino, about seven miles from UCLA's Westwood campus. She stayed with me for about a month and, in that time, she fell in love with Southern California. She made it clear that she wanted to go to college in the LA area, and like any doting father, I was so happy to hear that, and I told her I'd help her achieve her goal.

My move to UCLA was one of the most important decisions I've made in my career. In addition to my successful research program, I deliberately sought and developed a satisfying career in teaching students. When I began as a professor in 1985, I attended the medical school lectures in pharmacology, which is a required course for second-year students. I noted that the class was only half full, and many of the students in the room were either sleeping or reading the newspaper. Students would either show up ten minutes late, leave ten minutes early, or both.

The students clearly did not appreciate the way the course was being taught. One morning, just before the start of a lecture, I noted a stack of typed notes on the desk of a student sitting beside me. I asked her where she had gotten the notes. She told me that all of the students were getting their notes from the pharmacology course taught at the nearby University of Southern California (USC) School of Medicine. What a "kick in the head" to UCLA!

Several weeks into the course, I went to see the department chair, Don Jenden, and asked him if I could be given the opportunity and responsibility of becoming course director the following year. He promptly stated his concern that if I were to spend so much of my time teaching students, my research program could suffer. He reminded me that I had been recruited to UCLA due to my highly productive research. He also reminded me that I'd only been at UCLA for a few months, and that it was critical to launch my research program quickly and efficiently, without distraction.

"Instead," he suggested, "why don't you just give a few lectures in the course? That wouldn't detract appreciably from your important research."

"I assure you, I would never sacrifice my research for anything, including teaching, but I do have a passionate desire to teach medical students."

"Yes, but directing and running an entire eighty-hour course would be a gigantic commitment," he said. "You won't have any time to direct your basic research ... No, give a few lectures and be done with it."

It became evident to me why the pharmacology course was not very good; namely, the chairman did not give a damn about teaching.

I reminded him that the students had rated the UCLA pharmacology course as the worst-taught course in the medical school for many consecutive years and that this reflected poorly on him.

Well, that shut him up.

A few hours later, in the hallway, Don Jenden approached me and said that he would give some thought to my request. After several days of consideration, he came to my office and asked me to become course director for the next academic year.

My first year as course director worked out well. I had delivered about half the lectures (forty-two out of eighty) myself and asked a few other faculty who I knew to be good teachers to give the remaining ones. But I prepared all the questions for all the exams, and I graded all 150 myself. Now, that took time!

At the end of the course, the medical students rated Medical Pharmacology as the best-taught course in the medical school and gave me the "Golden Apple Award" for best teacher in the first two years of medical school. This teaching award is sponsored by the American Medical Student Association (AMSA) and is decided solely by the medical students, without any input or influence by faculty. This was an incredible honor for me to be recognized by my own students in this special way.

Don Jenden learned about this accolade and congratulated me. He could not get over the fact that I'd turned the pharmacology course around, 180 degrees, from the worst to the best, and in my first attempt.

Ironically, he asked me if he could give a few lectures in the course next year.

"Oh, so you want me to direct the course again next year?" I chided. We chuckled a bit, and I told him that I'd welcome his participation. I went on to direct the pharmacology course for twelve more years and received the Golden Apple Award each and every year.

Despite the time spent on my teaching profession, I wasted no time recruiting personnel and establishing a productive research program. Fortunately, my laboratory director at Tulane University, Keith Wood, had agreed to move to LA with me, and he did a fabulous job in getting our new lab up and running. We moved into my lab at UCLA in May, and we were conducting our first experiments on the West Coast by mid-August—a lightning-fast transition.

Between May and August, I scooted around the biochemistry, physiology, and chemistry departments at UCLA to learn more about the procedures I wanted to use to isolate, stabilize, and characterize EDRF, I hoped, as nitric oxide. During that short period of time, we ordered a top-quality recording spectrophotometer and an industrial chemiluminescense detector, both of which I needed for our critical upcoming experiments.

Paul Boyer, who had taught me enzymology and biochemistry in graduate school at the University of Minnesota, moved on to UCLA shortly after that, where he became professor of biochemistry and chemistry. The knowledge I had gained from him in graduate school was instrumental in my successful characterization of the enzyme guanylate cyclase. One day, I went over to his office on campus and introduced myself, explaining that I'd been one of his students in Minnesota in 1963 where I'd taken his Enzymology I and II courses.

"How did you like Enzymology?" he asked.

"Your Enzymology course was superb but one of the most difficult courses in the curriculum," I said. "But I wanted you to know that what you taught me enabled me to fully characterize the kinetic properties of the enzyme I was working with."

"And what enzyme might that be?" Paul asked.

"Guanylate cyclase, which catalyzes the conversion of GTP to cyclic GMP. Moreover, the molecule nitric oxide activates the enzyme several hundredfold and alters the binding affinity of substrate for enzyme."

"That's a fascinating subject, and I'd love to discuss more with you in the near future. Perhaps you can tell me about the kinetics of enzyme activation by a nitric oxide. That must be very interesting indeed."

I thanked him and left, pleased that I'd established a peer-to-peer connection with him.

I'd had ample experience with spectrophotometry from my research at Tulane Medical School. At Tulane, we had used spectrophotometry in experiments studying the reaction between NO and various forms of hemoglobin and guanylate cyclase.

Part of our experimental design was to perfuse a small segment of endothelium-intact artery with physiological salt solution. A small aliquot of perfusate (the fluid dripping out of the end of the artery) was quickly added to hemoglobin solution and analyzed by spectrophotometry. Any EDRF produced by the endothelial cells would wind up in the perfusate and, if EDRF was NO, subsequently react with the hemoglobin solution to form nitrosyl-hemoglobin, which has a red color. Adding acetylcholine to the perfusion solution would be expected to markedly increase the formation of EDRF and also the formation of the red-colored nitrosyl-hemoglobin. A few seconds after the acetylcholine was added, samples of the perfusate were added to hemoglobin. My eyes were fixed on the spectrophotometer.

I felt my heart pounding in my chest. I tried to picture what the spectral pattern should look like if the experiment were a success. The spectral pattern had to look like, or at least partially resemble, that obtained with the nitrosyl-hemoglobin.

I held my breath and watched as the spectral pattern changed sharply to match that of a known sample of authentic nitrosyl-hemoglobin. There was no pattern for hemoglobin. Only nitrosyl-hemoglobin was evident.

My heart rate climbed even higher. The experimental results were astonishing beyond belief. Acetylcholine stimulated the production of nitric oxide from the arterial endothelial cells. I realized in that instant that only one substance in nature could have caused such a shift in the spectral pattern, and that it had to be nitric oxide. This experiment indicated clearly and unequivocally that EDRF is NO!

Finally, I thought. *Finally!*

Everyone in my laboratory was ecstatic over our discovery. It was not possible to contain such information and jubilation strictly to the laboratory, and the news spread throughout the medical school. All of my students, postdocs, technicians, and fellows wanted to party. But first, I insisted, we had to conduct a few additional experiments in order to tidy up all ends and leave nothing to conjecture.

The conclusions based on the data observed were straightforward and unequivocal. EDRF and nitric oxide are one and the same chemical substance. We had proven by chemical means that EDRF is NO. Finally, my frustration had come to an end. Finally, we could say publicly that EDRF is NO. Finally, no one had to use the symbol EDRF anymore; it could be changed to NO. The schematic in Figure 7 illustrates this point.

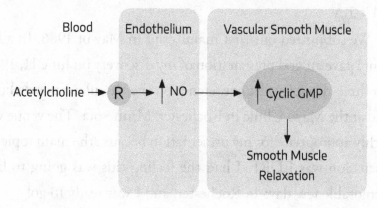

FIGURE 7

Our discovery revealed for the first time that mammalian cells could produce the gas nitric oxide. More importantly, in view of all of the known pharmacological effects of NO, we could now appreciate that such effects are operating "physiologically" in mammals. That is, NO production by arteries could arguably lower the systemic blood pressure and improve local blood flow through organs that require more oxygen and nutrients on demand (skeletal muscle, heart, brain). It could also prevent stroke and myocardial infarction by inhibiting platelet aggregation, as well as other effects. I felt that this was a provocative discovery with obvious benefits to humankind. At the time of our discovery, I realized that many investigators might soon enter the field of NO research and uncover many additional physiological effects of this unique molecule.

In view of the heated competition in this scientific field where many labs were trying to identify EDRF, we quickly wrote up our findings for publication and presentation at key cardiovascular conferences in 1986, only one year after my move from Tulane to UCLA.

We submitted our first manuscript in May of 1986. In addition, I gave an oral presentation of my discovery on June 11, 1986, at a three-day scientific conference on the Vascular Endothelium, held at the Mayo Clinic in Rochester, Minnesota. The venue was highly appropriate for my presentation because the main topic for discussion was EDRF. I had the feeling this was going to be a memorable few days in Rochester, and I was ready to go!

When it was my turn to speak, the moderator of the session, Professor Paul Vanhoutte, called me up to the stage and introduced me. I thanked him and looked out to the audience of about five hundred scientists. The auditorium was packed.

I started off with: "Ladies and gentlemen, today I am going to reveal the chemical identity of Endothelium-Derived Relaxing Factor or EDRF."

I paused because of the audience's reaction—lots of loud "oohs and aahs." When the noise subsided, I resumed my lecture.

"I am not going to reveal EDRF's identity immediately. Instead, I want you to listen to my entire lecture. At the end of my talk, I'll reveal the identity of EDRF, but I'm certain by that time, you will have already figured it out."

Suddenly, the auditorium went so silent that I could hear the people in the front row breathing. My forty-minute presentation culminated with the revelation that EDRF is NO, and what followed was a standing ovation accompanied by cheers.

When I opened the floor to questions, it seemed like everyone in the auditorium raised their hand at the same time. Fortunately, the session moderator fielded the questions for me.

Right at the start of the discussion, I noticed someone near the back of the hall, slightly to my left, stand up and rush out of the room. The gentleman was Professor Salvador Moncada from the London area. I wondered why he'd left so abruptly, and I hoped that he would return and ask some questions. He was a prominent investigator in the area of vascular pharmacology and EDRF. But he did not return. It was many months later that I learned from someone working in his laboratory that he had exited the auditorium to call his lab to inform them that EDRF is NO and that they should jump on this without delay. And they did. Salvador Moncada's group published the first paper to confirm our discovery that EDRF is NO.

Although I was hungry and ready for lunch, it was difficult for me to eat because I was bombarded with questions about my lecture. Indeed, I spent the entire afternoon talking with what appeared to be nearly everyone at the conference. But that did not bother me one bit. I was relieved that our discovery was officially public knowledge, and I was excited that finally, I was able to talk about it in public!

Several of my close colleagues and friends suggested that, after dinner, we all go to one of the local pubs near the Mayo Clinic. I seconded that suggestion.

The interior of the pub was built of dark wood, including the bar itself and the beams in the ceiling. The structure did not have many windows, probably designed to weather the many cold winter months in Minnesota. A small group of about ten or twelve of us entered the pub and walked over to the bar. There were too many of us to fit around a table, and we knew that by the time everyone arrived, we'd end up with a small crowd of about twenty-five.

As we began chatting, we were joined by others, many others, who quickly clustered around the bar. A few of my friends congratulated me on our discovery. I called to the bartender and announced that I would buy the first round of drinks. But my friend Bob Good quickly interjected and said, "No! Absolutely not! Lou is not paying for a single drink tonight. The first round is on me."

After a few drinks, our discussion picked up volume, which was interrupted by occasional applause. As the drinking picked up, the technical questions about methodology decreased sharply, and we talked more about how important this molecule could be for normal physiology. After all, nitric oxide was a new player on the block. Because it is a naturally occurring molecule in the body, we knew that the well-known pharmacological effects of NO are likely also to be "physiological" effects, that is, effects produced naturally by endogenous NO.

This revelation opened up new doors for physiologists to study exactly how NO regulates cardiovascular function. Most of the conference attendees were vascular physiologists and pharmacologists, many of whom also had been in the hunt for the identification of EDRF.

Then some of my colleagues began poking fun at me.

"Hey, Lou," one colleague said. "Remember when you told us that nitric oxide could never exist in biologic tissues because of its chemical instability and reactivity with other molecules? What changed your mind?"

In answering his question, the first thing I said was, "Never say never." And then I went on to say, "We decided to ignore the well-known chemical properties of NO and think outside the box, for a change."

On that comment, the group erupted with loud cheers and someone ordered another round of drinks.

One of my colleagues, Professor Phil Kadowitz, reminded me of the time, just a couple of years prior, when it was difficult for researchers to obtain funds from the National Institutes of Health and the American Heart Association to study the vascular effects of NO. Many scientists who were reviewing grant applications had questioned the merits of spending funds, government or private, to study a molecule that was a toxic gas in the Earth's environment. I nodded with the understanding that this was about to change.

"Now that NO has been shown to occur naturally in mammalian cells, it should be much, much easier to secure funding to advance our knowledge of NO. When you folks return to your offices, you should start writing and submitting research grants on the physiology of nitric oxide."

Then I added, "Nitric oxide is not just a gas "Blowin' in the Wind."

That comment triggered more cheering and still another round of drinks. Then, someone started chanting, "Bob Dylan, Bob Dylan," and the inebriated group quickly erupted into song.

My good friend, colleague, and organizer of the present conference in Rochester, Professor Paul Vanhoutte, was excited about our finding. He said to the crowd, "Tonight, nitric oxide is the most famous molecule in science. Now that we understand that EDRF is NO, we can all move forward and explore the physiology and pharmacology of NO."

Those comments by Paul brought more cheers. And more drinks.

By this time, the drinks were taking their toll on all of us, and I made the motion that we all retire for the evening because we had to continue with the conference at 8:00 a.m. the following day. That motion was seconded, and I slept very soundly that night.

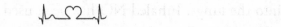

Our findings on nitric oxide opened up more opportunities to submit research grant proposals and raise funds to support our basic research program. Most of the funding came from the NIH, and other support came from the American Heart Association. At this point, we had more funds than we needed to take our research efforts to new levels. This was in sharp contrast to the grave situation we were in just six or seven years earlier when we could neither obtain grant support nor publish our work because the reviewers felt NO was not physiologically relevant. Ironically, those early, unpublishable studies led to the present discovery that our bodies produce NO. Now, *that's* physiologically relevant.

I tell my graduate and medical students all the time: never give up. Pursue what you believe in. Don't allow any temporary defeat to cloud your mind or interfere with the pursuit of your goals.

In 1994, the School of Medicine completely renovated and enlarged my laboratory into one big enough for twelve to fifteen people to work comfortably. A large, beautiful office was constructed adjacent to my lab, which served, among other things, to make visitors comfortable when they came to chat with me, as well as to hold small conference meetings with students and faculty. In 1996, I was honored with an endowed Chair in Medical Research from the Jerome J. Belzer, MD Foundation. One year later, I was given the title of Distinguished Professor of Molecular and Medical Pharmacology at UCLA.

Beyond our lab at UCLA, our studies quickly led to an avalanche of findings that nitric oxide produces a multitude of regulatory and beneficial health effects. NO facilitates cellular communication by diffusing across cell barriers from one cell into another and signaling all cells in its path. The overall role of nitric oxide in physiology is unique in that this molecule serves not only as a signaling molecule but also as a protective one. NO protects us against a wide array of aches and pains, illnesses and diseases. It raises sexual desires and athletic performance, lowers blood pressure, protects our skin from sun damage, and protects us from infection—the nitric oxide our bodies produce is as versatile as it is ubiquitous. No other single molecule in the body can provide all of these essential and beneficial effects.

Since NO is a gas, mixtures of NO and oxygen can be inhaled into the lungs. Inhaled NO has been used to dilate pulmonary arteries in newborns and infants born with life-threatening pulmonary hypertension. Babies born with constricted pulmonary arteries, resulting in inadequate oxygen exchange in the lungs, are visibly blue in color, but shortly after treatment with inhaled NO, their constricted arteries become dilated, and the babies turn pink. This therapeutic procedure was developed by Warren Zapol, MD, at the Massachusetts General Hospital in Boston, and it has saved hundreds of thousands of infants' lives.

Our original finding that mammalian cells produce NO led other investigators to take on determining how this comes about. One group, led by Professor Solomon Snyder at Johns Hopkins University, discovered that NO is produced from the amino acid L-arginine. This reaction was found to be catalyzed by an enzyme, which was appropriately termed NO synthase (this enzyme catalyzes the synthesis of NO from L-arginine). The details of the biochemistry of NO production were worked out by several investigators who went on to become prominent in their fields. Others discovered new actions of NO in different regions of the body. The field exploded, and publications on NO shot up from a few dozen in 1986 to several thousand by 1990. No other field of medical science had ever witnessed such an explosion of interest.

Answering one single question, *What is EDRF?* created a multitude of additional questions to be answered. I derived great personal satisfaction in following the basic research of many other investigators who were taking advantage of our original findings and extending them to so many different areas of physiology and biochemistry. This discovery was an excellent example of how basic biomedical research progresses from one fundamental discovery to another. I wanted to jump on this bandwagon because

I wanted to unravel a great deal more about the mysteries of NO in our bodies. Finding that EDRF is NO was not the end of our research endeavors. It was only the beginning.

Chapter 12:

Erectile Function and the "Father of Viagra"

I t was a sunny Monday morning in January of 1990 when Dr. Jake Rajfer walked down to my office. Jake was a professor in the Department of Urology at UCLA, in the same wing as my laboratory and office. We had known each other since I took my position at UCLA five years earlier. Academically, we didn't have much in common, as he was a urological surgeon, and I was a pharmacologist. But we enjoyed talking about other matters and often met for coffee in the cafeteria.

"So, Lou. Do you know what causes penile erection?"

This question caught me off guard. "I beg your pardon, Jake? Surely you jest!"

"Really, do you know what the neurotransmitter is that causes penile erection?"

"Okay, that's better. I'm neither a urologist nor a neuroscientist. I have no idea which transmitter is discharged from the nerves that attach to the erectile tissue. But you should know."

"The neurotransmitter is not known, and I'm wondering what kind of molecule it might be. Do you have any ideas?"

"Sorry, Jake. As I said, I'm not a neuroscientist, but I will give it some thought, and we can discuss this during our next coffee break."

"Okay. But before I go, let me ask you something. Is it possible that the neurotransmitter could be cyclic GMP? You've shown that cyclic GMP is a vasodilator. Penile erection occurs when the blood vessels in the penis dilate, and blood flows into the corpus cavernosum (erectile tissue)."

"Well, cyclic GMP is a vasodilator. You are correct. But it's produced inside the smooth muscle cells and acts inside the cells. When a neurotransmitter is discharged from a nerve, it travels into a small space, the synaptic cleft, outside the nerve cell and then interacts with receptors on the membrane surface of the adjacent target cells. There's no evidence to support any extracellular effects of cyclic GMP. It's strictly an intracellular signaling molecule. It's made inside the cells to act inside the cells."

"I see," said Jake. "But please give it some thought anyway, and we can talk about it next week."

I didn't give it any more thought that day. But the following day, it irked me that such an important neurotransmitter had not yet been identified. Down I went to the UCLA biomedical library to do a literature search on the subject. Within twenty minutes of reading, I saw clearly that what Jake had said was correct. The neurotransmitter responsible for penile erection was unknown. Not a single clue existed as to what it might be. Then I turned my attention to the physiology of penile erection, hoping I might gain some insight. Although I learned a great deal about the corpus cavernosum and how it becomes engorged with blood to cause an erection, I couldn't find any clues about a possible neurotransmitter.

Then I had a thought. What kind of nerves connect to the erectile tissue? Perhaps such information might give me a hint. According to most neuroanatomists, the nerve pathway to the erectile tissue should release acetylcholine, a well-known neurotransmitter. But that wasn't the case. The neurotransmitter was unknown. This was puzzling to me. As I continued reading, I learned that a urologist in Spain, Dr. Saenz de Tejada, had recently characterized the neurons innervating the corpus cavernosum but could not identify the neurotransmitter.

Fine, I thought. *Now I know all about the neurophysiology of the penis.* But that didn't get me very far along in trying to understand what the neurotransmitter could be. I began to get frustrated, and I argued with myself that I shouldn't waste my valuable time trying to figure out what neurotransmitter causes penile erection. Let the urologists and neuroscientists figure it out for themselves. Jake and I met for coffee a few days later.

"Well, Lou. Did you figure out what causes penile erection?"

"Yes. I know very well what causes penile erection, but I don't know which neurotransmitter is involved."

"Very funny, Lou!"

"I spent over eight hours reading and reading, and all I know is that the neurons are NANC nerves. The neurotransmitter remains completely unknown. I'm sorry I can't be of any help to you."

"Are you absolutely certain that it can't be cyclic GMP?"

After pausing for a few seconds of thought, I said, "I'm positive it can't be cyclic GMP."

We walked out of the cafeteria together and went our separate ways.

A few days later, while reading the latest literature on nitric oxide, I came across an article published by a neuropharmacologist who was also a good friend of mine. John Garthwaite, working at University College London, had discovered nitric oxide to be a neurotransmitter in regions of the brain having to do with memory and learning. This was the first time that NO had been identified as a neurotransmitter. At about the same time, Sol Snyder's group at Johns Hopkins revealed that neurons in the brain contained NO synthase, the enzyme responsible for the production of NO. And so, it made lots of sense that neurons possess the capacity to produce nitric oxide as a neurotransmitter.

Then came the epiphany! As I continued to read Garthwaite's article, I focused on his conclusions that certain neurons in the brain do NOT release acetylcholine. Instead, Garthwaite postulated that nitric oxide was the neurotransmitter.

"Oh my God! That's it. That's it!" I repeated out loud. If NO is the neurotransmitter in those special neurons in the brain, why couldn't it also be the neurotransmitter in similar neurons innervating the erectile tissue in the penis?

Without delay, I ran up five flights of stairs to the Urology Department and stormed into Jake's office. He had just emerged from surgery and sat down behind his desk.

"Lou, it's great to see you again. Why are you sweating? Here, sit down and relax for a moment, and then we'll go down and get some coffee. I need a boost after my last patient."

"I can't wait for coffee. I need to tell you something that you'll want to hear."

"Well, don't let me stop you."

"The neurotransmitter causing penile erection is nitric oxide! That's right. NO!"

After sitting back in his stained-wood, leather-bound reclining chair, with his hands behind his head, he said, "NO? How could it be NO? Isn't NO a gaseous molecule?"

"Yes, NO is a gas, but that does not matter because it's also soluble in aqueous media, just like oxygen. Oxygen doesn't work as a gas; it works in solution in the blood and tissue fluids. The same for NO; it works in solution in nerves, endothelial cells, smooth muscle cells, and so on."

"Go on ..."

"Do you remember when you kept asking me if cyclic GMP could possibly be the long-sought-after neurotransmitter?

"Yes, of course I do."

"Well, think about it," I said. "How does NO actually produce its effects in the body? That is, does NO work all by itself, or is some other molecule involved?"

"Oh, I see where you're taking this, Lou. You think that NO is the neurotransmitter, and NO elevates cyclic GMP levels in the corpus cavernosum to cause penile erection?"

"Exactly, Jake!"

"Oh my God! Oh my God!"

"That's exactly what I said to myself ten minutes ago."

This encounter was yet another perfect example of the Louis Pasteur phrase, "Chance favors the prepared mind." Pasteur used this statement in the nineteenth century to describe his remarkable ability to invent and innovate across a complex set of problems. He was a very learned scientist with an enormous knowledge base. In my career, I have found all along that the more knowledge I assimilated, the better my chances were of making original discoveries. One of the many exciting things about biomedical science is that the prepared mind can often provide clues even before performing any experiments.

Jake and I met for several hours during the week and planned our basic research approach to ascertain whether nitric oxide was the neurotransmitter responsible for erectile function. By combining our efforts, I knew we had a great chance of achieving success. My laboratory personnel had the expertise in studying isolated tissue preparations in tissue chambers and also measuring cyclic GMP levels and NO production in tissues. Jake and his residents were urological surgeons trained to implant prostheses into the penises of males with erectile dysfunction.

We all enjoyed a great camaraderie among the people from both teams. Before performing the planned experiments with human tissue, we chose to study rabbit tissue to establish the proper setup and experimental conditions. Human tissue availability was scarce, and we did not want to waste any in setting up our assay and working out the bugs, which are always inherent in any biologic assay. Once we were satisfied that our experimental setup was optimal, we began to experiment with human tissue, which Jake and his team supplied.

To implant a prosthesis in the penis, a relatively large portion of the corpus cavernosum had to be excised to make room for the implant. Usually, the excised tissue was discarded. But not anymore. A member of my lab team was always on standby just outside the operating room on days when such surgeries were scheduled. The attending resident would take the freshly removed corpus cavernosum tissue, place it in cold physiological salt solution, and exit the OR to give us the tissue. The tissue was then promptly brought into my laboratory for study.

Studying isolated erectile tissue was somewhat similar to isolated arterial segments. The principal difference between a setup involving corpus cavernosum and that for arterial segments is that the nerves within the erectile tissue must be stimulated electrically in order to cause relaxation and become engorged with blood. That's because in humans, rabbits, and other mammals, penile erection occurs as a result of stimulation or excitation of the nerves attached to the erectile tissue. In the absence of nerve stimulation, an erection does not occur, which is a good thing.

Experimentally, tiny electrodes were placed on either side of the tissue, and a small electric current was applied. This resulted in prompt relaxation of the tissue, as displayed on a polygraph recorder. The objective of our experiments was to determine what neurotransmitter is released from the nerves upon nerve stimulation to cause relaxation. I called a meeting involving the people in my lab and Jake's lab who we had assigned to work on this project.

"You all know the objective of these upcoming experiments. A few years back, some of you were also involved with the critical experiments leading to our discovery that the endothelial cells in arteries produce nitric oxide. Now, we are going to work with neuronal tissue within the corpus cavernosum to determine what neurotransmitter is responsible for penile erection. This is an incredibly important question; I'm sure you would agree. Keep in mind that there are no drugs currently available to treat the many millions of men globally who suffer from erectile dysfunction. The reason for that is simple. We don't know how stimulation of penile erection comes about. In other words, if we don't know what makes it work, how can we fix it when something goes wrong? But, by performing certain critical experiments, we have a damn good chance of changing that!"

Peggy Bush, one of my newest graduate students, and Georgette Buga, a research assistant with lots of experience testing isolated organ preparations, initiated the first series of experiments, which worked very well. Electrical stimulation caused relaxation of the tissues. These observations indicated that our experimental setup was operating the way it should.

"Okay, ladies. What should we do next?"

Peggy had a brilliant idea. "How do we know that the electrodes are not directly causing the smooth muscle to relax? That is, the electrodes may be touching the smooth muscle tissue instead of the nerves distributed inside the muscle. We want to be certain that tissue relaxation is attributed solely to nerve stimulation rather than direct muscle stimulation."

"Great point, Peggy. So how do we discern that?"

"Let's add a chemical compound that's known to paralyze nerves and prevent neurotransmitter release without affecting the smooth muscle."

"Excellent idea. Let's do it," I said.

The experiment worked. The complete blockade of relaxation indicated that electrically driven relaxation was mediated by the nerves scattered within the tissue.

"So far, so good," I said. "Now what?"

Georgette offered a logical suggestion. "Let's do the same thing we did for our successful experiments where we showed that EDRF was NO. Let's measure the tissue levels of both cyclic GMP and cyclic AMP to see if one or both are elevated during electrically stimulated relaxation."

"What will that tell us?" I asked.

"Both cyclic GMP and cyclic AMP are signaling molecules inside smooth muscle cells that cause relaxation in response to extracellular stimuli. Knowing if the production of one or both of these signaling molecules is increased upon nerve stimulation will give us a clue about what the neurotransmitter could be."

"That's an excellent explanation. Thank you!" I added.

The data were quite revealing. Electrical stimulation of the corpus cavernosum caused marked relaxation, which was accompanied by a sharp rise in cyclic GMP levels. On the other hand, cyclic AMP levels remained unchanged.

At our next lab meeting, Keith Wood, one of my longtime research assistants, suggested that we determine whether electrical stimulation causes a cyclic GMP-dependent relaxation. "An increase in cyclic GMP levels does not necessarily mean that cyclic GMP was responsible for the relaxation response. Maybe cyclic GMP was doing something else at the same time."

"What do you have in mind, Keith?"

"Let's do the same kind of experiments that we performed when we were trying to determine whether EDRF was NO. If we add a compound that inhibits cyclic GMP production, then relaxation should also be inhibited if cyclic GMP is involved in the relaxation process."

We did the experiments and found that electrical excitation of the corpus cavernosum caused cyclic GMP-dependent smooth muscle relaxation.

I called a lab meeting together and stated the importance of the data we had just obtained. Then, I was about to propose an experiment that we absolutely needed to do next. But before I got a chance, Peggy Bush approached me and asked if this project could be her basic research project for her PhD dissertation. "Great timing," I said. "Yes, of course. It's all yours! But now *you* will have to lead the way forward."

I started our lab meeting by saying, "Since cyclic GMP is obviously required for electrically mediated smooth muscle relaxation, nerve stimulation must be releasing a chemical that activates guanylate cyclase. Right? We already know from previous experiments on EDRF that NO can be produced by cells to activate guanylate cyclase and elevate cyclic GMP levels. Therefore, it's conceivable that the nerves in our smooth muscle preparations are capable of releasing NO. Let me ask you: What is a good, indirect way of determining whether the nerves are releasing NO?"

Georgette recommended that we test the effects of an inhibitor of NO production. I asked her to elaborate her thoughts for the group.

"NO synthase is the enzyme responsible for the production of NO in blood vessels. NO synthase has also been shown to be present in nerves in the brain, where NO can be formed. If NO is produced by the nerves in the erectile tissue that we are studying, NO synthase must be responsible for that production. Adding a known inhibitor of NO synthase should block NO formation and inhibit smooth muscle relaxation."

"Great explanation, Georgette. Okay, let's plan to do those experiments next. And once again, we need to measure not only smooth muscle relaxation but also cyclic GMP levels in the smooth muscle. If NO is indeed the neurotransmitter, the inhibitor should block both cyclic GMP formation and smooth muscle relaxation."

We conducted the experiments and the data were consistent with what we had expected. Inhibiting NO synthase activity abolished both cyclic GMP accumulation and smooth muscle relaxation. This was our strongest evidence so far that the nerves discharge NO upon electrical stimulation.

At our next lab meeting, I reviewed our up-to-date findings and asked Peggy for recommendations as to which experiment we should do next.

Peggy took the floor. "We've just shown in separate experiments that blocking either NO or cyclic GMP formation also blocks relaxation. What if we do the opposite regarding cyclic GMP? That is, what happens if we add a chemical compound that's known to magnify or amplify the actions of cyclic GMP without affecting NO? Wouldn't such a compound also magnify the relaxation response?"

"Great idea, Peggy. Let's test your hypothesis right away."

Once again, I took the time to explain to the group exactly why it was instructive to conduct such an experiment.

"Keep in mind that, physiologically, cyclic GMP is not only produced in response to NO but is also rapidly degraded and inactivated shortly after it is produced. The reason is that a signaling molecule, of which cyclic GMP is one example, should remain around for only a few seconds after it's formed. A longer duration would produce a greatly exaggerated physiological response, which is almost always undesirable. Cyclic GMP is rapidly inactivated by a specific enzyme termed phosphodiesterase."

After seeing a bunch of nodding heads, I went on.

"Having said this, what do you suppose the result might be if you added a phosphodiesterase inhibitor to the tissue baths in our experiments just prior to electrical stimulation?"

Peggy volunteered to answer my question, but I stopped her. "Not you, Peggy. You already know the answer. And this is your PhD dissertation work. How about someone else?"

Georgette gave a lucid answer. "The phosphodiesterase inhibitor should magnify both the increase in cyclic GMP levels and the smooth muscle relaxation in response to nerve stimulation."

"Perfect," I responded. "And if we are fortunate enough to get those experimental results, will that tell us anything about the possible chemical nature of the neurotransmitter?"

All hands went up, and with a YES response.

"And all together now. What would the neurotransmitter be if our experiments with the phosphodiesterase inhibitor work as you think they might?"

The unanimous response was, "NO!"

"Well, there's only one way to find out. Let's do the experiment!"

In the lab meeting that followed, I noted that everyone had big smiles on their faces.

"Why are you all smiling?" I asked. Peggy took the floor. "All the data we've assimilated thus far are completely consistent with the hypothesis that the neurotransmitter causing penile erection is our good friend, nitric oxide."

Then, both Georgette and Keith warned, "Before we can say that for certain, we've got to identify the neurotransmitter chemically as NO. We've already used chemical assays in the past to identify EDRF as NO. Let's just use the same assays to determine whether the neurotransmitter is also NO."

"Okay gang. This is it! Every single experiment that you've performed during the past few months has yielded data that are consistent with our hypothesis that the neurotransmitter responsible for penile erection is nitric oxide. Now, it's time to turn this hypothesis into scientific fact."

The experiments worked like a charm. We observed an eight-fold to tenfold increase in NO levels in electrically excited tissues compared to unstimulated controls. In a separate series of experiments, we tested the NO synthase inhibitor and found that it blocked the formation of NO.

At our weekly lab meeting, I congratulated everyone for making one of the most important discoveries of a lifetime.

"Do you folks realize what you have accomplished?"

"Yes," said Peggy. "I have a PhD research thesis to write."

"That you do. But let me explain my thoughts on all of this. You've discovered that NO is the principal neurotransmitter that causes penile erection in rabbits and in man. This physiology probably applies to many other mammals as well. By making this discovery, you've added a new dimension to the field of neuroscience by establishing that a gaseous molecule can function as a neurotransmitter. Your findings leave wide open the possibility that NO is a neurotransmitter in many other organs. You've also revolutionized urology by establishing the possible cause of erectile dysfunction. That is, a deficiency in the production of neurotransmitter NO. I'm certain that many research investigators in urology and pharmacology will jump on our coattails and attempt to synthesize a new drug for the treatment of erectile dysfunction."

Then it was Peggy's turn. "What kind of new drug? How might it work? What would its mechanism of action be?"

"Peggy, you tell us. After all, this basic research is your PhD dissertation. PhD signifies Doctor of Philosophy, so let's hear some philosophy."

"Well, one way, I suppose, might be to develop a drug that increases NO synthase enzymatic activity to make much more NO. Another approach would be a drug that amplifies the action of NO or cyclic GMP in the erectile tissue."

I cut in and said, "Both approaches sound reasonable. We're just going to have to leave it up to the urologists and neuroscientists to figure that out. We've done enough. We have established the foundation or building blocks for their future work. That's not so bad, is it?"

Peggy and I prepared a manuscript for submission to the journal *Nature*, which was considered to be the most prestigious and widely read scientific journal because most of the publications featured novel discoveries in nature. It was also the typical periodical for publishing important discoveries in the biomedical sciences. In the manuscript, we highlighted our finding that nitric oxide was the long-awaited neurotransmitter mediating erectile function. Further, we explained that this new knowledge could lead to the development of the first orally administered drug to treat erectile dysfunction, which afflicts 10 percent of the male population globally.

One week after submission of our manuscript, we learned that *Nature* rejected our work for publication. Moreover, we were told that our manuscript was not even sent out for peer review. Instead, the editor dismissed our work as unpublishable. The editorial board indicated that the members did not believe a gaseous molecule like NO could possibly function as a neurotransmitter. Yet, we provided incontrovertible evidence that NO functioned as a neurotransmitter. It was obvious to me and my research group that their evaluation of the merits of our work was flawed by their bias. No scholarly scientific journal should ever decide about suitability of any discovery for publication without first obtaining the opinion of at least two or three outside peer reviewers who are experts in the field of study. The editors of *Nature* were not experts in either neuroscience or urology.

After consulting with Jake Rajfer, we decided to submit our work to the *New England Journal of Medicine*. I had never published an article in that journal before and hoped that the editors of the journal would be more objective than those of *Nature*.

We received good news. Our work was accepted for publication without having to make a single revision and was published on January 9, 1992. Obviously, the editors of the *New England Journal of Medicine* saw merit that was apparently not visible to the editors of *Nature*.

The news media closely follows recently published articles from certain key medical journals, the *New England Journal of Medicine* being the most prominent. On the morning of publication, I received many telephone calls at my UCLA office.

The first call was from one of Larry Flynt's assistant editors of *Hustler* magazine. He asked if I would be willing to conduct a brief interview with him on penile erection. I paused for a moment as I assessed the possible consequences of such an interview. What kind of article would appear in *Hustler*, I thought? Then, it dawned on me that my mother was still alive and doing well. What if one of her friends would ask her why her son was featured in *Hustler* magazine? I respectfully declined the interview.

The second phone call was from an editor named Sandra Blakeslee at the *New York Times* newspaper. That interview request I accepted immediately. Sandra gave an excellent interview, and we spoke for about thirty minutes as I explained the significance of our work. She kept asking me whether nitric oxide could be used as a drug for impotent males to correct their erectile dysfunction. On several occasions, I attempted to explain that NO is an unstable gas that cannot be used as a drug to treat impotence. But I did add my opinion that biotech and pharmaceutical companies will soon begin drug development programs to come up with a drug that will enhance the effects of NO in the penis.

As I walked into my office to find some peace and quiet, an administrative assistant from the department office came to see me. She asked me if I had seen the article that had just been published in an Italian newspaper, *Repubblica*, which covered our recently described work in the *New England Journal of Medicine*. I told her that I had not, whereupon she gave me a photocopy, which included the cartoon illustrated in Figure 8. The cartoon was a vivid one, illustrating a man sitting in bed with his lady. Strapped to his back was a nitric oxide gas tank, and his lady had a big grin on her face.

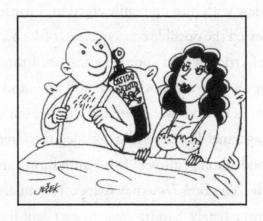

FIGURE 8.
THE WORDS ON THE TANK, "OSSIDO D'AZOTO" SIGNIFY
NITRIC OXIDE (OXIDE OF NITROGEN) IN ITALIAN.

A picture is certainly worth a thousand words.

The telephone calls continued throughout the day, and by evening, I was totally exhausted but pleased that our discovery received so much public attention. I wondered what the editors of *Nature* thought about all this newsworthy information.

The magnitude of our discovery was apparent. Several months later, the distinguished scientific journal *SCIENCE* published an article reviewing our work and declared nitric oxide as "Molecule of the Year."

Six years later, in March of 1998, I was sitting in front of my TV, watching the five o'clock news, when I heard the newscaster say, "We have breaking news about a newly approved drug for impotence." I literally jumped out of my chair and stood as I listened to the broadcast. Pfizer pharmaceutical company had just received approval by the FDA to market the drug *VIAGRA* for the treatment of erectile dysfunction in men. But that's all the information that was reported. My heart was racing.

I tried calling two colleagues at the New York City Pfizer office, but all lines were busy. I tried looking up information using my computer. Back in early 1998, the Google search engine had barely been established, and I did not know anything about it. Instead, I used two search engines popular at that time: AltaVista and Ask Jeeves. I learned that the generic name for the Pfizer drug was sildenafil, with the trade name of Viagra. After further reading, I came across what I was looking for.

The mechanism of Viagra was inhibition of a phosphodiesterase enzyme that inactivates cyclic GMP. By inhibiting this enzyme, cyclic GMP rapidly accumulates when NO stimulates its production. Therefore, Viagra works by increasing the effects of cyclic GMP and NO.

What made me feel so valued and validated was that the Pfizer research team reproduced our experimental findings and went on to develop a new drug on that basis.

The next morning, I went upstairs to see my urologist colleague, Jake. He had also heard the news and was elated to see me. "Now look what you've done! Congratulations!"

"Jake, we did this together. Neither one of us could have done this alone. That's what teamwork in science is all about. Do you realize what we have done for the hundreds of thousands of impotent men worldwide?"

"You mean tens of millions of impotent men," he corrected me. "Lou, do you remember when our first study on all of this was rejected for publication by *Nature*? That rejected work resulted in the marketing of Viagra. How do you suppose the editors feel now?"

"Frankly, I don't give a damn. But we can be certain that the editors of the *New England Journal of Medicine* feel proud and important."

"The good news is that we've done something truly great in medicine," Jake said. "But the bad news is that we had nothing to do with the development of Viagra. Therefore, we're not going to make a penny on Pfizer's sales."

"That's okay, Jake. Viagra is going to make you the most famous urologist in the world, just wait and see."

"That may be true, but my income is going to drop substantially."

"How do you mean? I don't understand. You should get a tremendous boost in your salary, not a decrease."

"It doesn't work that way in academic medicine. In addition to a fixed salary, I get paid by the number of patients I see for surgery. As you know, I see patients with erectile dysfunction and implant prostheses into their penises. My patients were unable to have sexual intercourse until I gave them life. And now, with the advent of Viagra, it's just a matter of time when I won't be doing this kind of surgery anymore."

"Oh, I understand. But still. Look at what we've done for these patients going forward. Don't you agree that they will be most delighted to take a pill rather than an implant?"

"Of course. I'm sorry to sound negative. Actually, I am quite proud of what we've accomplished."

We gave each other a big hug, and I walked back downstairs.

$$\sim\!\!\Omega\!\!\sim$$

Most pharmacologists and urologists recognized that the basic research in my lab made it possible for Pfizer to develop the concept all the way to the marketplace with Viagra. Consequently, I've been given the nickname: "The Father of Viagra." To this day, when I am invited to speak at a banquet dinner or conference, I am often introduced as "The Father of Viagra." I don't mind such a reference one bit. In fact, I find it kind of humorous. My mother, however, was not happy about it. She would get upset whenever she heard that phrase and would say to me, "Son, why don't you tell them to stop that already?"

The news about Viagra broke in March. Just seven months later, the Nobel Prize in Physiology or Medicine was announced. The date was October 10, 1998, a Monday. The prize was for the "Discovery of Nitric Oxide as a Widespread Signaling Molecule in the Cardiovascular System." Three scientists shared the Nobel Prize: Robert Furchgott, Ferid Murad, and me.

After recovering from the shock and excitement brought on by this announcement, I began thinking about the dates for the release of Viagra and the announcement of the Nobel Prize. I was struck with the timing of the two. The Nobel Prize announcement came only a short time after Viagra appeared on the market. *Was this a coincidence,* I thought, *or did Viagra play an instrumental role in persuading the Nobel Committee to consider NO?* After a few hours of investigation into the members of the Nobel Committee for Physiology or Medicine, I discovered that the majority were men over the age of sixty!

Chapter 13:
Sharon Elizabeth Williams

When I was teaching my Medical Pharmacology class at UCLA, I made a habit of going to the lecture hall about thirty minutes early each morning to organize my notes and write key information on the front board. One day, in October of 1993, I was preparing to teach when I noticed a female student walk into the lecture hall about twenty minutes early, take a seat, and begin to study.

The next morning, the same thing happened. I saw the same student walk into the hall, take a seat, and start studying. After some minutes of hesitation, I walked up to her and asked her why she liked to come to class so early.

She responded, "Good morning, Professor Ignarro. I live in Pasadena, which is about an hour's drive to the campus, but the driving time is so unpredictable because of traffic that I drive in early. First, I have coffee in the cafeteria, and then I come to the lecture hall to study a bit prior to the lecture."

"Good idea. This way you are not under much pressure, and you can relax before classes commence. By the way, what is your name?"

"Sharon Williams," she answered. I noticed she appeared to be about ten or fifteen years older than the average student in the class and was very attractive.

"I hope you are enjoying my class, and I want to wish you the best of luck."

Sharon continued to walk into class early, every morning, without missing a beat.

My style of lecturing involves looking directly at each of the 150 students in class while lecturing. Over the years, I've found that such an approach gets the students to pay closer attention to what I am saying. However, I began to realize that my eyes tended to linger more on Sharon than anyone else. I forced myself to gain control of my emotions and pay equal attention to all students in the class.

One morning, I walked downstairs to the Student Affairs Office, inquired into Sharon's date of birth, and learned that it was October 28. *Ah*, I thought. *That date falls on one of our pharmacology lecture days, which is coming up in a few days.*

October 28 fell on a Thursday in 1993. I walked into the lecture hall, as usual, about thirty minutes early. Normally, I am perfectly calm and relaxed before every lecture. I always feel so comfortable with my students. But not this one.

It was about 7:40 a.m., the usual time for Sharon to make her entrance. But 7:45 passed, and there was no Sharon.

Perhaps she decided to stay home, I thought, although she had not missed a single class since the semester started in August. Our class would begin at 8:00 a.m. sharp. I paced back and forth, waiting for Sharon to make her routine early entrance. It was now 7:55, and still no Sharon.

Then, my eyes lit up. Sharon finally made her entrance. I was about to wish her a happy birthday, but there were too many distractions. Students were chatting with her, and the classroom was noisy. I waited for an opportunity, but 8:00 a.m. struck, and it was time to start my lecture. As I stood up by the lectern, the class rapidly quieted down; not even a whisper could be heard.

"Good morning, class."

They were all looking at me. Then, while staring directly at Sharon, I whispered softly, "Happy birthday, Sharon."

She smiled broadly, and the students sitting next to her poked some fun at her and said, "Did you hear that? Dr. Ignarro wished you a happy birthday!"

Her smile made my day.

About six weeks were left in the course. Once the semester ended, I would not be seeing Sharon in lecture halls anymore. Although I had developed a strong desire to ask Sharon out for coffee or lunch, or simply to meet her in the cafeteria for breakfast, the better part of me said, "No way! She's a medical student, and I'm a professor who teaches one of her classes! Approaching her for a date would be totally inappropriate." And that's the way I determined it would remain for the next two-and-a-half years, at which time she would graduate.

Two long years went by without ever running into Sharon. In January of 1996, I received a telephone call from a good friend and colleague from Massachusetts General Hospital (MGH) in Boston. Professor Warren Zapol was chairman of the Department of Anesthesiology there. It was one of the leading anesthesia departments in the US.

Warren told me that a medical student at UCLA had applied for a residency program in anesthesia and that he was interested in recruiting that person to his program. I asked Warren for the student's name.

"Sharon Elizabeth Williams," he said. "Do you know her?"

After pausing for a moment, with all sorts of thoughts spinning in my head, I replied, "She was one of the best students in my pharmacology class."

"Yes, I know that. That's why I want her to come to MGH."

Warren asked me if I would contact her and try to convince her to do an anesthesia residency with him at MGH.

Great, I thought. *This is my path to seeing Sharon once again.* I promised Warren that I would speak to her right away. I did not have Sharon's phone number, so I decided to write her a note and leave it in her medical school mailbox.

The note said: "Dear Sharon. Do you remember me? I certainly remember you! Would you come to my office at your convenience? I want to talk to you about the anesthesia residency program at MGH," signed "Lou Ignarro."

The next morning, I heard a knock on my office door. I opened the door and there she was—a smiling Sharon Williams, wearing a white coat and looking like a real doctor.

We exchanged pleasantries, and, as my heart rate started to settle down, we had a chat about the anesthesia program at MGH. I told Sharon how well I knew Dr. Zapol, that he was a superb anesthesiologist and department chairman, and that he really wanted Sharon to join his program. Sharon said she was interested in the program and would give it serious consideration.

That was the last time I saw Sharon until her graduation, about five months later. I made it a point to go to the graduation ceremony and the reception that followed in the garden area just outside of Royce Hall on campus. My intention was to congratulate Sharon during the reception, but she was surrounded by classmates, friends, and family members, and I felt out of place and uncomfortable crashing her party.

Oh well, I thought. *I'll just wait a couple of weeks and then try contacting her. Perhaps she would agree to have coffee with me sometime.*

About two weeks later, I ran into one of Sharon's classmates in the hallway and asked her for Sharon's contact information. I told her I wanted to talk to Sharon about the status of her pending residency program. I was told that all she knew was that Sharon had moved back to the East Coast to begin her internship in the Washington, DC, area. Upon hearing that, I thought I might never see Sharon again.

Although it was difficult and sometimes painful, I tried to keep Sharon out of my thoughts and just keep moving forward. In the back of my mind, I planted the idea that I would contact my colleague Warren Zapol at MGH in a year or so and try reaching Sharon through that route, assuming she had selected his residency program. A few months later, just as I was beginning to move Sharon to the back of my mind, another one of her classmates came to my office early one morning to talk to me. Mihaela Balica told me, point blank, "Dr. Ignarro, I think you should go out with my friend Sharon Williams."

After a long pause, I said, "What? Why do you say that?"

Mihaela continued, "Because I remember the way you paid attention to Sharon a few years ago in the pharmacology class. I think you should go out with her."

There I was, wondering what brought this on and why Mihaela cared about my asking Sharon out. Then I thought that perhaps this was all Sharon's idea to send her friend to plant the seed and get things rolling. And so, I asked Mihaela if Sharon knew anything about this, and she said absolutely not. Mihaela insisted this was her idea and that Sharon was unaware of our meeting or discussion.

"If you think I should ask Sharon out on a date, you need to tell me how to contact her, because I don't even know where she is right now."

"No problem. Here's her telephone number in Virginia, where she's living right now with her mother. Why don't you call her? It just so happens that Sharon is planning to fly to Los Angeles in a few months to take a short vacation, and she will stay with me at my place."

She handed me a piece of paper with Sharon's phone number, already prepared. I thanked her very much and promised her I would call Sharon in a few days. As Mihaela walked away, I stared at her and wondered what had just transpired. *Did this really happen?* I thought. *I actually have the opportunity to see Sharon again. It's not over yet.*

Later the same afternoon, one of my laboratory assistants, Georgette, walked into my office. This time, it was not about any experiment in the lab. Instead, Georgette said to me, "My friend Mihaela told me she came by to see you this morning about dating Sharon Williams, one of your former medical students. I think you should date her, too."

"Georgette, what's going on here?" I said. "You are the second person today who thinks it's a good idea for me to ask Sharon out. What did Mihaela tell you about Sharon and me? Please share that with me. I have no idea what's going on."

"Mihaela told me that you singled out Sharon in class to wish her a happy birthday." Georgette continued, "You must be interested in her. Mihaela and I just feel that Sharon is good for you, and you should see her again."

"But Georgette, how do you know that Sharon will agree to see me again?"

"Trust me, I know she will."

With that, Georgette went back into the lab. I did not know what to think anymore. But one thing was certain. I would call Sharon the next day.

The next afternoon, I tried calling Sharon. However, she was not at home, and I left a message to call me back with the excuse that I was curious about her decision regarding the anesthesia residency program. She returned my call the following evening.

We spoke briefly about her internship at Washington General Hospital, and I asked if she was also living in our nation's capital.

"No, but I'm living nearby in Alexandria, Virginia, with my mother. My father passed away recently, and I wanted to stay with my mom during this difficult period."

"Oh, I'm so sorry to hear that. It must be difficult working as a busy intern and also taking care of your mother."

I told Sharon that I was calling to inquire about her decision regarding her upcoming residency. I reminded her that Dr. Warren Zapol was pressing me to convince her to select his program at MGH.

Sharon understood that. "I have not yet decided, but I will do so very soon. I am also considering the anesthesia program at Johns Hopkins Medical Center in Baltimore, which is also an excellent program. Moreover, Baltimore is a lot closer to my mom than Boston."

"I understand fully." Then I asked her a rhetorical question. "Sharon, are you planning to come to Los Angeles anytime soon?"

"Yes, I am. I am flying to LA to see my close friend, Mihaela Balica. Do you remember her from class?"

"Yes, I do. In fact, I got your phone number from Mihaela because I wanted to call you about the residency program."

"Oh, I was wondering how you found my number."

I asked her when she would be coming to LA and discovered she'd be in town in late February, just a couple of months away.

"Do you think we could get together for coffee while you're here?"

"Yes," Sharon responded. "I'd like that very much."

Oh! That was a great answer!

I wished her well and said bye for now. Then I sat down in my chair and realized that I was sweating. *That was some phone conversation*, I thought. I put my hands behind my head and started to daydream about seeing Sharon once again.

About two weeks prior to her visit, I started to count down the days to her arrival. Before Sharon, I was never nervous about having a date with a woman, even if it was just for coffee. On the day after her arrival, I called her. Mihaela answered the phone, and I asked to speak with Sharon. "Good luck, here she is," Mihaela said.

We exchanged pleasantries and did a little catching up. During our conversation, I came up with the idea of asking Sharon to dinner instead of merely for coffee. *Here goes*, I thought.

"Sharon, would you like to join me for dinner while you are in town?"

She paused for a second or two and finally said, "Yes, that sounds like a plan."

"Great, I know that you are here only for a few days. So, how about tomorrow evening?"

"No, I'm sorry, but I am busy tomorrow night."

Feeling dejected, almost rejected, I asked her if she would be available the following evening. This time, she said yes.

Fantastic! I thought. *I've got a real date with Sharon Elizabeth Williams!* I'd dreamt about this day since the fall of 1993, nearly four years prior, and now it was finally happening.

The date was March 2, 1997, a warm and sunny Sunday. I could see that I would arrive about ten minutes early, so I decided to drive around the block a few times before I knocked on the front door. But as I approached Mihaela's home in Brentwood, I looked out and saw Sharon standing outside, waiting for me.

She's also ten minutes early and waiting for me outside on the sidewalk. What does that mean? I thought. *Is she anxious to see me, too?* I was about to find out.

I pulled my car up to the curb and walked over to greet her. She looked absolutely stunning. I gave her a hug and said how great it was to see her again.

I walked her over to my car and opened the door for her. We drove off, and I explained that we were going to Santa Monica to dine at Ivy at the Shore, on Ocean Avenue. She liked that idea because, although she had never eaten at that restaurant, she enjoyed seafood. We began our conversation by talking about her internship in Washington, DC. It was a grueling position, as she had to work about one hundred hours each week.

Unbelievable, I thought. The conversation then changed to her pending residency in anesthesia.

"Have you decided where to do your residency?"

"Yes, Doctor Ignarro, I have."

"Please call me Lou. You are a doctor now, as am I."

Sharon continued, "I have decided to go to the Johns Hopkins program in Baltimore because it's only an hour's drive to my mom. I want to be close to her since my dad recently passed away. I hope that your friend Dr. Zapol is not too upset with me. I called him to explain my choice."

"Warren should not be upset at all. I'm certain that he understood the situation. Sharon, you did the right thing, and I'm sure your mom is pleased with your decision."

As we began eating our dinner, we found so many topics to talk about. One thing I noticed was that neither one of us was eating that much. Normally, I don't let anything get in the way of my meal in a great restaurant. But I simply could not eat. I had no appetite, although I was starving before I picked up Sharon. Looking across the table, I saw that Sharon was not eating much either.

"Sharon, don't you like the cuisine here? You are not eating."

"Yes, the food is delicious. I just don't have much of an appetite. But I don't see you eating much either. Is the fish okay?"

"The fish and everything else is very tasty. It's just that, for some reason, I don't have much of an appetite either."

We continued to talk as we sipped on chardonnay but without eating much more. I asked her if she would care to walk around outside a bit before I took her back to her friend's home, and she agreed. We walked up and down Ocean Avenue and also to the Santa Monica Pier. The weather was perfect and warm for an early March evening, and the sound of the breaking waves was romantic.

On the way to Mihaela's place, I asked Sharon if we could get together the next evening. *This is the second big test,* I thought. *She agreed to our first date, but will she agree to a second date, on the very next evening?* I anxiously awaited her response.

"I'm busy tomorrow night. Mihaela and I made plans to get together tomorrow night after she gets off work. I think I need to do that with her."

As I was preparing what to say next, Sharon asked, "What about tomorrow afternoon? Do you have time to go to the movies in the afternoon to see the new *Star Wars* movie?"

I was relieved and responded, "Yes, of course. Great idea. I want to see the new release, too."

The next day, I parked in my spot at UCLA, and we walked over to the theater in Westwood to see *The Empire Strikes Back.* Although it was an exciting film, I was distracted by sitting so close to the lady by my side. Throughout the movie, I contemplated slowly reaching over and gently touching her hand, but I chickened out every time. I knew I had only five days before Sharon had to fly back to DC.

On the way to her friend's home, I asked Sharon out for the next evening. That would be three dates in a row. With a twinkle in her eye and an incredibly sexy smile, she said, "Yes, of course."

It was the "of course" part that jolted me, as if I had stuck my finger into an electric outlet. I suggested we go to dinner again but this time to an Italian restaurant, Valentino, in Santa Monica.

And then, I asked her if she had time in the late afternoon to go for a walk in Santa Monica before having dinner. She agreed to both, and I drove her home.

I am batting a thousand! So far, so good! But where am I going to take this? I thought. She had several years of commitment on the East Coast, with her internship and residency, and I was more than well established at UCLA on the West Coast. Then, I started asking myself one question: Where do I really want to take this? Do I want a short-term relationship, or do I want a long-term relationship? How could we have either one, as we would be living three thousand miles apart for at least several years? I stopped torturing myself by saying out loud, "Que sera sera!"

The next afternoon, I took Sharon for a walk along a path with beautiful views of the Pacific Ocean. The sun was beginning to set, and the orange sky in the west was magnificent. While walking, I reached down and gently grabbed her right hand with my left, waiting for her response.

She accepted my hand and squeezed it, turning around with a smile. We continued walking slowly without saying a word to each other. This should have been a relaxing moment, but I was too excited to remain calm. *The time is right,* I thought. I stopped walking and turned Sharon around to face me. Then I placed my hands on her shoulders, pulled her toward me, and kissed her as passionately as I could. I don't do anything halfway.

We stared at each other for a moment and then heard several distinct "wolf whistles" from a group of guys who had apparently observed Sharon and I kissing. We both laughed out loud and continued walking. Now, I felt relaxed. The pressure had dissipated, and I was starting to notice I felt hungry. My appetite had returned.

We drove to Valentino, where we ate delicious Italian cuisine accompanied by excellent red wine. Valentino is noted for their extensive wine cellar with a wide selection of Italian wines. During the meal, I asked her if she liked Italian cooking.

"Yes, I do. Italian food is one of my favorites, and this restaurant is fabulous."

"I'm glad you like it. You know, the next time you're in town, I'd love to take you to my mom's home in nearby Downey and have her cook an authentic Italian meal for us. She's such a fabulous cook that I call her a chef."

"I'd like that very much," she answered. "But that may be some time from now because I won't be able to take another break until I complete my internship in the summer."

"I understand. But we'll figure something out." A moment of silence followed. Then I continued, "Sharon, I need to drive to San Diego on Thursday because I've been invited to speak at a pharmacology conference on Friday morning. I'll drive back up to LA right after lunch. It's the annual meeting of the American Society for Pharmacology and Experimental Therapeutics, and I've been asked to give a special plenary lecture on my basic research."

"It must be on nitric oxide," she said.

"Yes, it is, and I'd like you to come to my lecture."

"Are you asking me to come with you to San Diego the day after tomorrow?"

"Yes, I am. I would like you to know something about my work, and I'd like you to meet some of my friends."

I did not expect her to agree to join me. But, after a short pause, she said yes. That made my evening.

We had a pleasant drive to San Diego, I introduced Sharon to several of my good friends, and then took her out to dinner.

This evening turned out to be special indeed! Sharon made me feel like no other woman had ever done. I'd not been able to get her out of my head since she arrived in LA a few days prior. I wondered what I would do when she left in two days.

We headed back to LA just after lunch.

"Sharon," I said, "what are we going to do after you leave for the East Coast tomorrow?"

"What do *you* want to do, Lou?"

"I want to see you again, and sooner than later!"

We agreed that I'd come out to DC and visit.

When we arrived back in LA at her friend's home, I gave Sharon a big hug and thanked her for the magnificent time we had spent together.

Two months later, in late April, I visited Sharon in DC. I stayed for a few days at a nearby hotel but saw very little of her. Her work in the hospital kept her busier than one can imagine. But we did get some quality time together, and I told her that I'd like to come to DC again, perhaps in the early summer. Sharon said that was fine as long as I understood how busy she would continue to be.

Several days after returning home from visiting Sharon, I realized that I could no longer be without her. The pain of separation was too much to bear. I called Sharon and told her I wanted to see her again in a few weeks.

On the flight to Dulles International Airport, I decided that I was going to ask Sharon to marry me. The date was May 31, 1997—my birthday! But I had not told Sharon it was my birthday.

Sharon had just finished being on call and drove over to my hotel. It was about 5:00 p.m. when she pulled up. I asked her to have a drink with me before we went out for a bite to eat. We sat down at the bar, and I was about to say something when Sharon looked straight into my eyes and whispered softly, "Happy birthday, Lou."

"Ahh, you remembered! Do you remember when, a few years ago, I whispered 'happy birthday' to you just as you entered the classroom?"

"Of course. How could I forget that? Look what it eventually led to."

"And what it might continue to lead to," I added. "Sharon, I'd like to make a toast, to us. Actually, I wish to pose a question to you."

"And what would that be?" she asked with an unforgettable smile. I think she knew what was coming next.

"Sharon, I love you very much! Will you marry me?"

Her eyes lit up, and she opened her mouth slightly but said nothing for a few seconds.

"Yes, Lou, I would love to be your wife."

I pulled her off the bar stool, nearly causing both of us to fall, and we embraced.

"Sharon, what a journey this has been."

She modified my remark and said, "What a *romantic* journey this has been."

"Okay, dear, let's get ready for dinner," I said.

"Lou, before we go to dinner, I want you to meet my mom. I'll drive us to Alexandria, about thirty minutes away, and then you and I can go to a nice restaurant in that area."

Her mom, Dorothy, was an energetic woman of eighty-four years of age. She had a great sense of humor and was happy to meet me. During dinner, Sharon insisted that I had to get her mom's permission before we could get married. I agreed. The three of us went to lunch the following day, and I politely requested permission to marry her daughter. She gave me a big hug and said of course.

On the last day of my brief three-day visit, we began planning our special day. Sharon considered all the possible options, keeping in mind her internship and the start of her anesthesia residency on July 1. There was no break in between. She said she could take her two-week vacation any time during her residency, suggesting that the end of July and beginning of August would be good.

Sharon did not want a big wedding. Instead, she preferred to elope but have a big reception following the wedding. We eloped to Las Vegas on July 30 and held our reception in Beverly Hills on August 2.

We were married in a tiny chapel in Las Vegas that was decorated with colorful plastic flowers and two tiny indoor waterfalls. Our limo was a 1959 pink Cadillac Eldorado, driven by a man with spurred cowboy boots. The minister's wife, who was in her ninth month of pregnancy, took photos as she rested her camera on top of her belly like a makeshift tripod.

On the way back to the hotel, Sharon said, "What have I done to myself?"

We both laughed and agreed that this had been an experience never to forget.

Our mothers, other relatives, and friends all were disappointed that we'd eloped, but they were exuberant at our reception three days later, on August 2, at an Italian restaurant in Beverly Hills. I had arranged to rent the entire upstairs of Prego Ristorante for that evening. Charles Shapiro, the restaurant manager, took especially good care of us. The food and wine were excellent, and everyone had a great time.

We had no desire to fly out of the country for our honeymoon. Instead, we both decided it would be fun to drive up the Pacific coast to Napa and Sonoma wine country, with an initial stop in Carmel-by-the-Sea for two days. The bed-and-breakfast establishments, restaurants, and wine tastings were all superb and romantic. This is what Sharon needed as a break away from her internship and residency and a chance to relax.

On the drive back, we planned to see one another throughout the next year, where I would spend half my time in Baltimore with Sharon and the other half by myself in Malibu in two-week stints. We would repeat this sequence for the entire year from August of 1997 to July of 1998. I set up an office in Sharon's home in Baltimore so I could easily communicate with my laboratory and the departmental office several times each day. Sharon was busy at the hospital from 6:00 a.m. to 7:00 p.m. every day, and I had dinner prepared and ready for the two of us each evening.

One evening at dinner, about halfway through the first year of her residency, Sharon asked me if I was okay with her completing her anesthesia residency in Baltimore. She was concerned about my frequent traveling between Los Angeles and Baltimore. I told her I was most definitely okay with the commute and that I wanted her to continue her residency in the best program in the country. Then she brought up an alternate possibility.

"What if I transfer my residency to the anesthesia program at UCLA?" she said.

"Would you do that? How good is the anesthesia program at UCLA?"

"Well," she said, "it's not as good as that at Johns Hopkins. But if I finish this first year here in Baltimore, I should be in pretty good shape to spend my second year at UCLA."

Deep down inside, I was ecstatic at this possibility, and I could sense my heart rate rising, but I did not want to influence Sharon in any way. The decision was up to her.

"That decision is up to you. I told you I don't mind traveling back and forth. I want what is best for you and your career."

"Thanks for your support, but I want us to be together all the time, not just for two weeks at a time. Don't you feel the same way?"

"Sharon, I love you very much. You are the love of my life. Of course, I would rather be together all the time. So, tell me, what are you going to do?"

She stood up, grabbed me, and said that she would arrange for her transfer to UCLA in six months. I looked into her eyes as my own overflowed with happiness, and I hugged her tightly.

PART IV:
The Nobel Prize

"Life is either a daring adventure or nothing at all."
— *Helen Keller*

Chapter 14:
Nobel Prize Announcement

At the time of Alfred Nobel's death in 1896, his worldwide business empire consisted of nearly a hundred factories for the manufacture of explosives and ammunition. Needless to say, Nobel had amassed a great deal of wealth. His will revealed a dramatic surprise for his family, friends, and the general public. He had always been generous in humanitarian and scientific philanthropies, and he was no different in death. He left the bulk of his fortune in trust to establish The Nobel Foundation that would come to be the source of the most prestigious of international awards, the Nobel Prizes.

Nobel's reasons for the establishment of the Nobel Foundation are unknown. However, there is speculation that he became disappointed and depressed every time he was criticized that his inventions with powerful explosives would inevitably lead to war and many deaths. He had a difficult time defending himself against such accusations. Perhaps he thought that establishing the prizes in his name, to be given to those who most benefited mankind, might clear the air regarding the destructive capability of his inventions.

In an excerpt of the will, Alfred Nobel dictated that his entire remaining estate should be used to endow *"prizes to those who …. shall have conferred the greatest benefit to mankind."* He established five distinct prizes: physics, chemistry, physiology or medicine, literature, and peace. There are now six distinct prizes. In 1968, Sveriges Riksbank (Sweden's central bank) established "The Sveriges Riksbank Prize in Economic Sciences in Memory of Alfred Nobel." Today, the prize in economic sciences is often called "The Nobel Prize in Economics," but it is not one that was in Nobel's original will and testament.

In addition to establishing the categories for the prizes, Nobel dictated two criteria that must be met for the prizes in physics, chemistry, and physiology or medicine. The first criterion is that the person under consideration has to have made an original discovery. Nobel did not intend the prize to be awarded to someone who expanded or extended the field; the person had to have *discovered* the field. The second criterion was that the discovery had to be of clear benefit to mankind. A discovery, no matter how provocative, without clear benefit to mankind, would be insufficient to warrant the Nobel Prize.

Perhaps the most popular category is the Nobel Peace Prize, probably because the individuals receiving this prize are well known worldwide. The Nobel Peace Prize is so popular that people often congratulate me for winning the Nobel Peace Prize instead of the Nobel Prize in Physiology or Medicine. That does not bother me, but what is rather disconcerting is when I am congratulated for winning the "Nobel Peace Prize in Medicine." Just think about that for a moment.

One morning, on Wednesday, October 15, 1997, I received a telephone call from our department chairman, Mike Phelps, that Paul Boyer had just been awarded the Nobel Prize in Chemistry. I quickly went online to the Nobel Prize website and saw that Paul shared the prize with two others for their pioneering work on the mechanism by which ATP is used by the muscles of the body for energy production. I walked over to the Molecular Biology Institute to congratulate Paul. He thanked me, but I could see that he was being bombarded with press coverage and TV cameras, so I left him alone and returned to the medical school.

Only three people at UCLA had received the Nobel Prize, and all were in chemistry. They were Donald Cram, Glenn Seaborg, and now Paul Boyer. No one had been awarded the Nobel Prize in Medicine at UCLA.

In May of 1998, twelve years after my initial discovery of nitric oxide, I received an invitation to go to the Karolinska Institute in Stockholm to deliver a lecture on my work pertaining to nitric oxide. The Karolinska Institute, the largest medical and research university in Sweden, and one of the most prestigious in the world, often conducts seminar programs where internationally renowned scientists are invited to speak on their basic research. I gladly accepted their kind invitation, and my lecture was scheduled for July, just two months later.

I arrived a few days ahead of time to visit two of my good friends and colleagues at the Karolinska, professors Jon Lundberg and Eddie Weitzberg. Jon and Eddie also worked in the field of nitric oxide and were interested in why our exhaled breath contains nitric oxide gas. We had met on several previous occasions at scientific conferences and often discussed our basic research.

I asked them, point blank, "Why does human exhaled breath contain NO?"

At that time, the clear answer had yet to be determined, but they offered the explanation that the NO in the airways (trachea and bronchi) causes the smooth muscle in the airway to relax, thereby facilitating bronchodilation, which enables breathing.

They also told me that elevated levels of exhaled NO might be a predictor for asthma. That possibly asthmatics produce more NO in their bodies' attempts to cause bronchodilation so they can breathe easier.

One highlight of my visit was taking an evening cruise on their twenty-foot motorboat through the canals in Stockholm harbor. The boat was equipped with an inboard engine and could seat up to about eight persons. The night's cool breeze was filled with soothing music, as my friends were not only talented scientists but also talented in the arts, and they played their guitars and sang Swedish folk songs. I had not felt so relaxed in a long time.

During the evening, Jon explained that my lecture promised to be very special in that it would be given in the auditorium within a building called the Nobel Forum, which houses the Nobel Committee for Physiology or Medicine, and where the committee meets to make the big decision of who will win the Nobel Prize. Eddie added that committee members often attend the lectures held in the forum.

Oh, I thought. *There goes my period of serene relaxation on this wonderful boat ride. I had better give the best lecture of my life.*

The remainder of the boat cruise, conversation centered on how I might present my research contributions. My friends Jon and Eddie told me to relax and just give the same kind of talk that they had heard me give before.

Easier said than done.

The following morning, I got up early and took a long, refreshing walk all around Stockholm, thinking about my lecture scheduled for later that afternoon. My friends picked me up at the Grand Hotel, and we headed off for the short drive to the Karolinska Institute. On arrival, I walked over to slide control and gave them my PowerPoint presentation. People began to trickle in, and then the pace picked up. I could see that the audience would be large.

Just before we were ready to begin the session, Jon came over to tell me that there were at least three Nobel committee members in the audience. He hastened to add that in the past, several invited speakers at the forum later went on to win the Nobel Prize.

"Oh, thanks, Jon, for informing me," I said with a touch of sarcasm. "That's a good way to get me to relax."

It was time to start. Jon introduced me, and I proceeded to the podium. After thanking Jon and welcoming the audience, I started to talk science. As I got into it, I began to feel calm and relaxed. I could see that I had everyone riveted to their seats. At certain key points in my lecture, I saw the Nobel committee members in the audience taking notes. Each time, I highlighted what I had just said to make my points even clearer.

The lecture came to an end after about forty-five minutes, and I'd covered all of the important points pertaining to my discoveries involving nitric oxide. When I finished, I received a standing ovation, making it clear to me that everyone enjoyed the talk. I felt great.

Then came the Q&A. Two of the three committee members in attendance raised their hands and asked me questions. Their questions were pointed and pertinent, and I believed that they must have read my published work.

After the Q&A, one of the committee members introduced himself to me and asked if I would step outside. I recognized him as the prominent cell biologist and histologist Professor Tomas Hökfelt, who used histochemistry (chemical approaches) to visualize the insides of cells. He grabbed my hand and walked me to a quiet corner of the building, in between two potted trees. It was clear to me the way he kept looking around that he did not want anyone to hear or even see us speaking to one other.

I had no idea what to expect. He was not smiling. Indeed, his facial expression was one of extreme seriousness, even concern. Then he leaned over to me, nearly touching my head with his. To this day, I'll never forget what he said. As I began to sweat, he asked me, "Do you believe that there is a Nobel Prize waiting for the field of nitric oxide?"

My sweat glands immediately poured sweat into my suit. *My God*, I thought. *Why is he asking me this? Is it because the medicine committee is thinking about awarding the Nobel Prize to the key investigators in the field of NO? Why else would he ask me that question?*

By this time, my heart rate had caught up to my rate of sweating.

"Yes sir, of course. I believe that nitric oxide is most worthy of the Nobel Prize."

As I was about to continue with a more detailed justification, he interrupted me, raised his tone of voice, and asked me why I felt that way.

I started to explain the universal role of NO in physiology, but he interrupted me again.

Once again, he looked all around the room to be certain no one was watching us converse. Then, he continued his interrogation.

This time he asked me what my major contributions to the field were.

I gave him my long list of contributions, one by one. This time, he did not interrupt me once.

As I finished speaking, he thanked me, shook my hand, and said, "Good work, and good luck!" And then he left. I was shaking like a leaf and ready to wet myself.

Jon and Eddie had witnessed this exchange, and as soon as I was alone, they came up to me and asked me what the hell we talked about for so long.

I said, "Okay, I'll tell you, but first let's go get a drink at the nearest bar."

We had to drive back into town to the Grand Hotel to find one. My friends felt that the Q&A after my talk in the forum went well. But they wanted to know more about my private discussion outside the auditorium. I explained everything that transpired, and we all agreed that this private encounter could turn out to be important later, if the NO field ever were to be considered for the Nobel Prize.

Announcement

The announcements for all Nobel Prizes are generally made during the first or second week of October, with the one in Physiology or Medicine being first, on a Monday. NO had been passed over for the prize year after year, so I had no expectation that 1998 would be any different.

During the second week of October in 1998, I was in Nice, France, to attend a scientific advisory board meeting for a small biotech company (Nicox) involved in developing nitric oxide-based drugs. On Monday the 12th, I was scheduled to leave Nice from the Côte d'Azur Airport to catch a short flight to Naples,

Italy, where I had been invited to spend a few days and give a lecture on my research to the School of Pharmacy at the Federico II University of Naples. It was a beautiful, sunny day in early October in Nice, so I went for a walk outside the hotel before heading for the airport. As I was walking along the coastal area adjacent to the beach, I had a feeling that today was going to be my lucky day. After all, I was headed to Naples, where my dad was born way back in 1896, and I always loved visiting.

I entered the airport in Nice and checked in to my flight to Napoli. While standing in line to board, an airport attendant walked by and said out loud, "Is there a Professor Ignarro here waiting to board? You have an important telephone call."

I panicked because the first thought that came to mind was an emergency back home. I signaled to the young lady who asked for me, and she handed me her mobile phone and told me to speak fast because we were about to board the flight to Naples.

I grabbed the phone from her and was surprised to hear that the person calling me was my good friend Dr. Robin Farias-Eisner. He calmly asked me how I was doing and how the weather was in Nice. The tone of his voice did not connote any kind of emergency or sense of urgency.

I abruptly cut in, "Robin, is there some sort of emergency at home or at the university?" I was expecting perhaps LA had been hit by an earthquake or that a large brush fire was burning out of control in Malibu, where I owned a home.

"No, not at all." His answer surprised me and left me wondering why he'd called. *How did he know that I am in the Nice airport waiting for my flight to Naples?*

Robin interrupted my line of thought and cheerfully explained, "Lou, I'm calling to congratulate you! Congratulations!"

"What the hell are you talking about, Robin? Congratulate me for what?"

Then he said, "Are you sitting down?"

"No, I'm not sitting down; I'm standing in line and ready to board my flight. It's really nice to hear your voice, but why are you calling me at the Nice airport, at 4:00 in the morning your time?"

"The announcement just came from Stockholm," he said. "You've won the Nobel Prize in Medicine!"

I paused for a moment, a long moment. I thought this was a bad joke. A very bad joke. Then I reasoned, *Why would my friend take the time and effort to track me down in an airport six thousand miles away at 4:00 a.m. his time just to pull my leg?* I did vaguely recall that the Nobel Prizes are usually announced from Stockholm at 12:00 noon on a Monday during early October, and it was indeed October 12.

My heart began to pound out of control. As I was about to further question Robin, the airport attendant yanked her phone back, saying, "I'm sorry, sir, but it's time to board the plane."

I pleaded, "Please, wait one more second, please!" I felt like she'd stripped off my clothes as well. No luck.

I boarded the plane in a state of total confusion and took my business class seat in the first row, wondering whether any of this was real or if I had just suffered a hallucination.

Not knowing quite what to do, I came up with a brilliant idea. I looked up and stared at each passenger who entered the plane as they walked by. I tried to get their attention so that they would look at my face. I figured that perhaps the Nobel Prize announcement made the newspapers, and perhaps my photo had been published along with the announcement. If that were the case, then maybe someone might recognize me. But, unfortunately, no one recognized me, and some probably thought I was a crazy man, the way I stared at them.

The plane landed smoothly at Capodichino airport and taxied to the deplaning area. Capodichino is a relatively small airport, so passengers must walk down mobile stairs to deplane then walk the tarmac into the airport terminal. As my plane approached the docking area, I looked out the window and saw hundreds of people standing on the tarmac, presumably waiting for our flight. I wondered why so many people were waiting for this flight to arrive. When the plane came to a complete stop and the seat belt signs were turned off, I stood up, grabbed my carry-on luggage, and proceeded to deplane.

Upon reaching the top of the stairs, I looked out in front of me and noticed dozens of camera flashes with all the people staring up at me. I wondered what all this fuss was about and reasoned that either the president of Italy or Andrea Bocelli must be standing behind me, so I turned around to see who was there.

Not seeing anyone special, I began to descend the stairs, and as I reached the tarmac, I recognized my close friend Professor Giuseppe Cirino from the University of Naples, who had invited me to come. Giuseppe, called "Pippo" by his friends, was a well-known pharmacologist working in the nitric oxide field.

"Pippo!" I said. "Do you always greet your friends this way?"

Pippo was sweating and with a giant grin, answered hastily, "Lou, Lou, did you hear the news?"

Since I was not positive "the news" I had heard an hour ago in Nice was true, I answered, "No ... what news?"

His grin got even wider as he showed me a piece of paper and told me to read it. But the language was Swedish. Nevertheless, I tried to read the document. In bold print was a lengthy Swedish word, **NOBELFORSAMLINGEN**. All I needed to see were the first five letters: **NOBEL**. Then, my eyes darted down the page where I recognized my name, ***Louis J. Ignarro***.

Both of my legs gave way, and I headed for the ground at high velocity. Several people came to the rescue, picked me up off the ground, and escorted me into the terminal.

I yelled as I gave Pippo a big hug.

Waiting inside the terminal was another close friend of mine, Professor Bill Sessa from Yale University, who also had been invited to Naples to give a lecture. Clearly, all my friends had heard about the Nobel Prize before I did. In fact, it appeared that the entire city of Naples had gotten the news. Several distinguished politicians, including the mayor of Naples and the mayor of Campagna (the region within which Naples is located) were present to greet and congratulate me. And all those people I saw standing on the tarmac and taking photos were local reporters who were there to interview me.

I was bombarded, literally attacked, by the press for interviews. After accepting a few brief interviews, I begged Pippo to please get me out of there. Pippo and Bill, as well as the police, shielded me from most of the other reporters and whisked me away to a nearby limousine, which the mayor of Campagna (Sindaco di Campagna) had arranged to get me to my hotel. The limo ride to my hotel was like none other I had ever experienced. A ride from Capodichino airport to the city center of Naples, which would normally take about forty minutes at that time of day, took only ten minutes by motorcade. Once again, I tried to focus on the Nobel Prize announcement but found it difficult to do so in a speeding limousine. The streets of Naples are not conducive to speeding, especially by oversized vehicles like limousines, and I found it truly amazing that we did not sideswipe any other cars or pedestrians.

As we approached our destination, I was told that my hotel had been changed and my room upgraded at no cost. Dozens of people greeted me upon entry into the hotel. The mayor presented me with gorgeous flowers and a dozen beautiful silk ties from the Marinella tie shop, located in the nearby Santa Lucia region of Naples. Then, we proceeded up to the hotel's rooftop restaurant for a cocktail party. The Italians sure know how to celebrate. The hors d'oeuvres and sparkling wines were fantastic.

The fact that I had just been awarded the Nobel Prize did not fully register in my mind until several minutes after being escorted to my private suite. The room was so quiet compared to the deafening noise of the preceding few hours. I sat down to rest before unpacking my suitcase, and that's when it hit me. *The Nobel Prize ... oh my God ... oh my God.*

As I sat in a most comfortable chair with my feet raised up on the ottoman, a glass of Chivas Regal in one hand, I began tracing the events of the day. Then I started to think back to a few months prior when I was in Stockholm to give a lecture on my basic research discoveries, which was followed by an interrogation by a prominent member of the Nobel committee. Now, I was convinced that I had indeed given the best talk of my life.

Which of my studies convinced the Nobel committee to award me with the prize? I kept running the question through my head. *Was it figuring out how nitroglycerin works as a vasodilator? Was it our discovery that EDRF is NO? Was it our discovery that NO causes penile erection, which led to Viagra? Was it all of the above?* It didn't matter to me. The only thing that mattered was that I had been awarded the Nobel Prize in Physiology or Medicine for my discoveries on nitric oxide.

I felt a strong urge to return home to celebrate with Sharon, my family, my students, and my friends. However, it wouldn't be right to leave Naples without giving my invited lecture to the students at the university. It would be a couple of days before I could return to the US.

The foundation always makes a point of informing the Nobel Laureates before telling the news media. This way, the Laureates receive the news from the most reliable source. In my case, Sharon and I had recently moved from Malibu to Westwood, so the foundation did not have my new number and was unable to reach me by telephone, thus I was informed by email. However, I had only recently purchased my first cell phone, and it did not have international coverage. Therefore, I left it at home. I was later told by members of the Nobel committee that I was the first Laureate ever to be informed of the prize by email.

As I started to unpack my suitcase, Pippo came to my room to assist me in contacting Sharon. After speaking with Sharon, I finished unpacking and sat down again to rest. As I began to reflect on the day once again, I was interrupted by Pippo, who burst into my suite and told me, "Put on a suit because we're going out to dinner! We must be downstairs in the lobby in fifteen minutes, please!"

"But Pippo," I protested. "We just ate and drank, and I'm tired."

He began pacing back and forth in my room and gesturing with his hands, as most Italians do. "No, I'm sorry, but we must do this. This is a special day for Italy and especially for Napoli."

As an Italian, I well understood the significance of this upcoming dinner.

"Okay," I told Pippo, "I'll be down in the lobby in fifteen minutes."

Again, we were escorted in a government limousine driven at high speed. The event included government officials, dignitaries, local scientists, and friends. I've always been fond of Italy's cuisine and wine. Every region of this beautiful country is proud of its local foods and regional wines, and I've never had a less than superb meal anywhere in Italy. But the cuisine in Naples is special to me, as it was the style I grew up with.

Pippo, Bill, and I began talking about the Nobel Prize and how I felt about receiving such an accolade, but we were continually interrupted by people who came by for photos and to congratulate me—so often that I found it difficult to savor, or even finish, my dinner.

Upon arriving back at the hotel, all I wanted to do was rest. My friends wanted to have a nightcap, but I begged them to let me sleep. I returned to my room and flipped on the TV, and the first thing I saw while scanning the channels was an interview with me that had taken place earlier in the day. There was no escape.

I set my travel alarm for 7:00 a.m. and attempted to get some sleep because I knew I would have a busy day ahead. But I could not sleep. Despite all the fabulous wine I'd had for dinner, I was flying high. Sleep was impossible. Jet lag was nonexistent. I felt like I should get up, go outside, and run a marathon. The stress, excitement, and emotion likely stimulated my adrenal glands to release large amounts of adrenaline and cortisol, all of which kept me excited and attentive. My only remedy was to begin walking in circles around my suite.

Despite the pressure from back home to return as soon as possible, I felt obligated to give my lecture as promised. And so, my friend drove me to the university to prepare for my lecture. The original invitation was for me to give a lecture exclusively for the School of Pharmacy. However, because of the news about the Nobel Prize, the venue was changed to include the entire university. I've never seen so many students and faculty together in one place. The audience was so large that additional rooms were set up with audiovisual accommodations so that everyone could "attend" my lecture.

Realizing that the audience would now include people who were not scientists and would not be able to understand my planned lecture, I revised my talk on the fly so I could speak in a way that would capture everyone's interest. Afterward, I had the opportunity to meet many students with diverse backgrounds. But they all had one thing in common: they wanted to take a photo with a Nobel Laureate.

Chapter 15:
Celebration after Celebration

F ollowing the event at the University of Naples, it was time for yet another dinner and another spectacular evening, after which I returned to my hotel, packed for my morning departure to LA, and went to bed. This time, I was able to get about three hours of sleep. My flight schedule had been changed so that I could return home a bit sooner than originally planned. But I was concerned because most flights within Italy leave late. The original plan was to be driven from Naples to Rome, a ninety-minute ride, and then take a flight from Rome to LA. I had always preferred that route because there were no connecting flights in Italy to worry about.

However, the revised plan was to fly from Naples to Milan and from there to LA. The potential problem was in making a timely connection in Milan. I checked in to my flight at the airport in Naples and was told that the flight was scheduled to depart on time at 10:00 a.m., with boarding time set at 9:30. So, I was at the gate at 9:30, ready to board. But no one was working at the gate. Then, 10:00 a.m. came and went and still—no one at the gate.

I started to worry, and I asked an airport attendant walking by, "Is this flight delayed? Why is the plane not boarding yet?"

He replied in broken English, "What time is the flight supposed to depart?"

I told him 10:00 a.m.

He looked at his wristwatch and said to me, "Ten o'clock, nine o'clock, twelve o'clock ... what's the difference? We leave soon."

It had taken me two days to get my heart rate down to near-normal, and that comment sent it spiking up again. If the flight left at noon, I would likely miss my connection in Milan and not get home until twenty-four hours later. I had to think of something, and fast. And then it came to me.

I was carrying the previous day's Italian newspaper, in which the front page had a clear photo of me at the airport on my arrival from Nice just after the announcement of the Nobel Prize. The headline read something like this: ***Premio Nobel Assegnato a Prof. Louis Ignarro***, which translates to ... Nobel Prize Awarded to Professor Louis Ignarro. I ran over to the gentleman who was so unconcerned about the time of day and showed him the front page of the newspaper. He looked at the photo, then looked at me, then looked at the photo again and said, "Oh mio dio! Sei tu!" *Oh my God, it's you!*

I seized the opportunity to say that this flight needed to board and take off as soon as possible, or I would miss my flight from Milan to LA. He jumped up and promptly organized the airport staff to board the flight. We took off fifteen minutes later, and I had plenty of time to make my connection. It's a good thing I had brought a copy of that newspaper!

The staff at the Malpensa Airport in Milan all knew who I was as soon as I deplaned the flight from Naples. A dozen people greeted me planeside and escorted me to the VIP lounge, where I was fed a nice lunch with red wine. Even the captain of the flight to LA showed up to congratulate me. He told me that although this particular Boeing 747 jumbo jet did not have first-class seating, he would assign me the entire front row of business class so that I could lie down on one side of the aisle and eat on the other side.

The captain also asked me what I would like to eat so that the staff could make arrangements before takeoff. You see, in Italy, it's all about the food. Just before takeoff, which was on time, incidentally, the flight attendant brought me a glass of cold prosecco together with a cheese plate. It appeared that the flight would be quite comfortable. I sat back, relaxed, and enjoyed the view over Milan.

After reaching cruising altitude, my rest was interrupted when the captain came by and invited me into the cockpit. Once he'd introduced me to the co-captain, navigator, and one other crew member, he asked if I was at all familiar with flying a plane. I told him the closest I'd come to flying a plane was playing with my Microsoft Flight Simulator, which has a Boeing 747 as one of many planes to simulate.

The captain said he thought that the Microsoft Flight Simulator software was quite realistic and then started to ask me all sorts of questions about the controls in the cockpit. I think I impressed him because I was familiar with the controls on the flight simulator. He advanced me to the co-captain's seat and went through most of the controls with me. He then asked if I was ready to take over the controls.

"Of course not! I've never flown any kind of plane before!"

"Yes, you can fly this jet," the captain said. "You won the Nobel Prize! You should be able to fly anything." He then made me grab the yoke, and, with a calculated smile on his face, he assured me not to worry. "The plane is flying on autopilot."

I was greatly relieved.

Back in the cabin, I enjoyed a delicious dinner with vino rosso (red wine) and was able to get some sleep for most of the flight. The descent and landing were uneventful, and once I'd gone through customs, there waiting for me were Sharon, my mom, some people from my laboratory, and a bunch of close friends. It was so good to be home, at last.

My mom had a special greeting for me. Instead of congratulating me, she reminded me that I first learned about winning the Nobel Prize when I was in Napoli. She added, "That's where your father was born, and that's not a coincidence. This was planned all along, and, if I were you, I would consider going back to church again."

The next day was another busy one, this time at UCLA. I had made this trip to France and Italy during the midterm break in the medical pharmacology course that I teach to the second-year medical students every year. I never had a break during any other part of the course because I was so deeply involved with it. The class met five days a week from 8:00 to 9:00 a.m. from mid-August to mid-December, for a total of sixteen weeks.

When I walked into my office at 5:00 a.m., I was startled to see it overflowing with flowers and plants. I was later told that they all had been delivered throughout the day of the announcement on the 12th. I had never before had so many flowers in my office. In fact, I'd never before had *any* flowers in my office.

When I walked into class, I received a long standing ovation and was given a large congratulations card (about three feet by two feet) with the signatures of all 150 of my students.

That made my day.

The students requested that, before I begin my lecture, I tell them two things. One, where and how I first learned about the prize, and two, how I reacted and felt after learning about it. My response, plus the Q&A that followed, took about twenty minutes, which meant that I had only thirty minutes remaining to give my planned lecture. But I figured that was okay. It's not every day that a professor gets the opportunity to explain to his class how he reacted upon learning that he was awarded the Nobel Prize.

After class, I walked back to my laboratory, where my graduate students, postdoctoral fellows, visiting fellows, and technicians all were waiting to congratulate me. They broke out singing, "For He's a Jolly Good Fellow."

I was deeply touched by this.

"It's all of you who should be congratulated," I said. "After all, you are the ones who did all the experiments, calculated all the data, prepared all the charts and graphs, and helped me write the manuscripts. Thank you all very much."

At that instant, I heard someone knocking on the lab door. I turned around and saw that it was Paul Boyer, director of the Molecular Biology Institute.

He stepped over and gave me a big hug. "Last year at about this time, you came over to congratulate me. Now it's my turn to congratulate *you*, my friend."

I thanked him for the kind words, and something suddenly came to mind.

"Paul, do you recall that you were my professor and teacher in graduate school many years back?"

"Of course, I do!"

"Well, I was just thinking that I am so glad you got the Nobel Prize before I did. It would have been awkward the other way around. The teacher should come before his student."

Paul laughed and, in his humble manner, said, "I'm lucky to win the prize at all."

I assured him that he certainly deserved the Nobel Prize for his far-reaching discoveries on cellular energy production. We then picked a date to have dinner together at the University Faculty Center, and he left to return to his office.

When I arrived back at my lab, my group explained to me how disruptive the last few days had been because so many people, including the news media, had come by looking for me. The local TV stations had come to interview me for the evening news, but they were told that I would not return from Italy for another couple of days. Nevertheless, my people were interviewed in my absence, and they did a fabulous job explaining what we had discovered over the years and its relationship to cardiovascular health.

One of my technical staff, Russ Byrns, was known around the lab for his sense of humor. Several months earlier, he had taken a photo of me standing on the floor near one of the laboratory benches, pointing my index finger toward my personnel as if to tell them to keep busy and not waste time. He was good at photography and had the photo enlarged to the size of a lifelike figure. He then printed a large caption above my head, reading **"Nobel Shmobel, Get Back to Work!!"** The TV news media loved it, filmed it, and it appeared on the evening news on three different networks.

At the time the interviews were occurring at UCLA, the news media found out where my mom was living in Downey and went there to interview her. Three of the major networks (NBC, CBS, and ABC) conducted the interviews. They had politely asked Mom if she would kindly conduct a TV interview, and she did not hesitate to say, "Yes, of course! I'm proud of my son."

But she made them wait while she brushed her hair and changed her clothes. Mom was eighty-four years old at the time and was totally with it. I later saw replays of the interview on one of the networks and was proud of the way she conducted herself. She was poised, relaxed, and funny as well.

Upon being asked about my childhood and what factors motivated me to want to go to college and then eventually be awarded the Nobel Prize, Mom explained how, at the age of only ten years, I built firecrackers and bombs and made rocket fuel. She also mentioned my interests in model railroads, what a good auto mechanic I was, and that I raced cars and brought home many trophies. She told the reporters that I was motivated in anything I set out to accomplish. All in all, Mom did a better job with the interviews than I could have done.

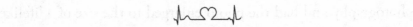

Just as things began to settle down, representatives of the Nobel Foundation began calling and emailing to plan for the Nobel festivities that would be held over a six-to-seven-day period during the first week of December in Stockholm. I had many tasks I needed to accomplish in the coming few weeks.

For example, I was obligated to find a tuxedo shop and get my exact suit measurements so that I could send this information to Stockholm, where the Nobel Foundation routinely uses a local tuxedo shop to prepare the white tie and tails for all participants in the Nobel Ceremony and Banquet. Then, I worked with the

Nobel staff to arrange our flights from LA to Arlanda Airport in Stockholm. After that, I was asked about all the guests I planned to invite to Stockholm. I was surprised and delighted to learn that up to twenty-five guests per Nobel Laureate could attend and participate in the Nobel Ceremony and Banquet. They wanted a detailed guest list. After I provided my guest list, the foundation provided Sharon and me with a tentative schedule of events for Nobel week. We could see that it would be a full week indeed.

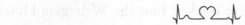

One evening, while relaxing in front of the TV and thinking about the events of recent weeks, I reflected on two dates in particular: the announcement of the marketing of Viagra, which came in March of 1998, and the announcement of the Nobel Prize in Physiology or Medicine for the discoveries pertaining to nitric oxide, which came just a few months later, in October. I had already learned that the majority of the committee members were men over the age of sixty, and I made the obvious connection. *Could this really be the only reason for my Nobel Prize?*

As I was to learn a few weeks later in Stockholm, my discovery of NO as a neurotransmitter that led to Viagra was not even considered in the decision of the Nobel Prize pertaining to nitric oxide. Apparently, only the basic research conducted up through 1986 was considered for the prize. This was about five years before our revelation that NO was the mediator of penile erection in humans.

Right about this time, I received a FedEx package from the White House. Wondering what it could be, I opened the large envelope to find a single sheet of paper. A letter of congratulations from President Bill Clinton, together with an invitation for Sharon and me to attend a special welcome party for the American Nobel Laureates of 1998.

The event was to be held in mid-November at the White House. I had never been inside the White House, so I was quite excited to have the opportunity to tour the interior. All seven of the Nobel Laureates were booked into the Watergate Hotel along the Potomac River, a short car ride to the White House. Of course, the Watergate was well known because it had been the headquarters of the Democratic National Committee in 1972, near the end of the first term of the Nixon administration. It was here that the infamous Watergate break-in occurred, engineered by Nixon's staff, to steal important files pertaining to the Democratic Party as they prepared for the upcoming presidential election. The Watergate Hotel also was where Ms. Monica Lewinski, one of President Clinton's aides, resided while working in the White House. The news of the president's affair with her had come to light in January of 1998, and the ensuing impeachment hearings loomed on the horizon.

At about 5:00 p.m. on November 24, we all gathered in the lobby of the hotel and waited to be driven to the White House. This was a good opportunity for the seven Nobel Laureates and their spouses to greet and get to know one another. I already knew Ferid Murad, Bob Furchgott, and their spouses, Carol and

Margaret, respectively, but I had not previously met the other four Nobel Laureates. In two separate vans, we were driven to the first of three security gates, where officials checked our passports and the contents of our pockets and purses, and they inspected any cameras we brought in. After two more security checks, we were finally escorted to the "Red Room," where guests would sit and wait until the president was ready to meet and greet them.

When the time came, we were escorted into a large gallery, where each Nobel Laureate was introduced to the president. Following the greeting of each Laureate, the president met with each couple before opening the event to everyone in the ballroom. One of the president's aides announced that the president would have limited time to spend with us because of other pressing issues, and then we all were escorted into the ballroom.

Exceedingly friendly and inquisitive, President Clinton was a delight to talk to. He asked each of us about our discoveries and how they impacted humankind. His queries made him sound more like a scientist than a politician, and no one brought up any policy issues. The president appeared to be relaxed and enjoying this rare moment away from the hassle of politicians and accompanying news media near the peak of the Lewinski scandal.

About thirty minutes into our interactions with the president, I was standing next to him when one of his aides approached and told him that he had to leave immediately to go to another meeting. President Clinton told him that he was not yet ready to leave this gathering, and that he would leave a little later.

The president continued asking each of us pertinent questions not only about our discoveries but also about scientific discoveries in general.

I waited for a pause in the discussion and then developed a dialogue focused on the limited availability of government funds to support basic biomedical research in the United States.

"Mr. President," I said, "I'm sure you already know that the great majority of American researchers in the biomedical field receive their funding from the NIH, right here in Washington."

"Yes, I am aware of that," the president said.

"Very importantly, sir, without those NIH funds, it is highly unlikely that I would be here in the White House as a Nobel Laureate, chatting with you."

President Clinton responded, "You and the other Nobel Laureates in this room should be very proud of our mission to support biomedical research, and research in all the sciences, for that matter. No other country does what we do for our scientists."

"I agree with you completely, Mr. President, but I want to add that we don't have quite enough funds to handle the growing number of young, bright investigators. We would all love to see an increase in the NIH budget."

My colleagues standing next to us agreed that the NIH was ready for an increase in its budget. In response to our plea, the president said, "I promise you that I will do what I can before my term is up."

I thanked President Clinton and, just then, the presidential aide came by again to fetch him.

The president told his aide to cancel the meeting because he wanted to stay right here in this room with us. Of course, we all were delighted he chose to stay.

The president then walked around the ballroom, stopping to chat with each of us individually. Sharon and I enjoyed the moment. He even let me use my own camera to take a photo of Sharon and him. I learned a great deal about our president in such a short time. Bill Clinton was charming, polite, and very knowledgeable in many areas.

Hillary Clinton was noticeably missing for most of the night. But then, toward the end of the evening, the Laureates were gathered together, and we were taken into a separate room. There, Hillary awaited us. Each of us was introduced to Mrs. Clinton, and we were asked to give a thirty-second summary of our scientific accomplishments in layman's terms. That was not an easy task, especially for the Laureates in physics, who tried so valiantly to explain their discovery of *"a new form of quantum fluid with fractionally charged excitations."*

I couldn't even understand what they were explaining.

When my turn came, Hillary took one good look at me while shaking my hand and said, "Oh, yes, aren't you the one who invented Viagra?"

We all laughed, and then I explained that my discovery of nitric oxide led to the development of Viagra by a big drug company, not by me.

She retorted, "Well, isn't that the same thing?" Clearly, she had been briefed about my role in the development of a drug that she probably didn't appreciate talking about at the time of this particular White House gathering.

Chapter 16:
Ceremony in Stockholm

When we returned home after a delightful experience at the White House, Sharon and I had about three weeks to prepare for our excursion to Stockholm for the Nobel festivities. Although we had no idea what to expect, we looked forward to the occasion with great anticipation. We departed Los Angeles on a warm and sunny day on December 4 and landed at Arlanda Airport in Stockholm on December 5 in a snowstorm. We were greeted planeside by a gentleman who knew me by name, but I did not know who he was at the time. He introduced himself as Professor Nils Ringertz, chairman of the Nobel Assembly. Professor Ringertz took Sharon and me to our waiting limousine. During the thirty-minute drive from the airport to the Grand Hotel, we talked about the Nobel Foundation and about my contributions to physiology and medicine. He was a prominent biochemist at the Karolinska Institute and had followed my research on nitric oxide. Professor Ringertz explained to us that we were in for an excellent time in Stockholm but warned that I would be busy for several days.

He also informed us that each Laureate would have his own personal and full-time limousine and chauffeur. Professor Ringertz then introduced our chauffeur as Hans, who was driving as we spoke. Hans would even stay available to my family when I was busy with official events. Sharon and I looked at each other and agreed that we were in for a grand time.

The limousine pulled up to the front entrance of the Grand Hotel. Working our way through the large, beautiful snowflakes falling from the sky, we were escorted by Professor Ringertz into the hotel lobby, where we were greeted by numerous smiling, yet unfamiliar faces of hotel and Nobel Foundation staff. One was a lady who introduced herself to us as Margarita. She was an employee of the Swedish State Department who was assigned to be our personal aide or attaché for the duration of the Nobel festivities. Margarita sat down with us for a few moments to explain our daily schedule. She was friendly, personable, and open with us, and explained her role to assist us with anything we needed. She looked very Swedish, with long blond hair and a fair complexion, standing about five feet, eight inches tall. Together, we walked through spacious hallways carpeted in blue and gold to our harbor-view suite directly in front of the hotel. Sharon and I unpacked and took the chance to rest in anticipation of a busy week.

Every morning, Margarita stopped by to review the schedule and go over the timing of each commitment with me. I did not have to carry the schedule with me or even remember what was coming next. She handled it all and made certain I didn't slip up.

Although Sharon and I could not spend every day and evening with our family and guests, we were able to have breakfast together every morning in the Grand Hotel. For my twenty-five invitees, I invited my mother, brother, daughter, Sharon's mom (Dorothy Williams), sister (Susie Cluff), and brother-in-law (Mike Cluff). In addition, we invited several persons who were graduate students in my laboratory (Peggy Bush, Michele Gold, Georgette Buga, Adrian Hobbs), as well as a few key figures at UCLA, such as the chair of Pharmacology (Mike Phelps), dean of the School of Medicine (Gerald Levy), and chancellor of UCLA (Albert Carnesale).

Also invited were two close colleagues of mine at UCLA. One was Robin Farias-Eisner, who was the first person to inform me that I had been awarded the Nobel Prize. The other was Gautam Chaudhuri, who'd worked with me in research and teaching since the first day I arrived at UCLA thirteen years prior.

At our first breakfast together in Stockholm, tables were lined up so everyone had a nice view of the harbor right in front of the hotel. The breakfast was a generous buffet with excellent coffee. We sat down at the table with all of our family members at about 9:00 a.m. I glanced over at my mom, and I noticed her looking at her wristwatch and shaking her hand up and down as if to check if the watch was working. I knew exactly what was on her mind.

"Mom, is something wrong with your watch?" I asked.

"Yes, the damn thing is broken again."

"Are you sure about that?"

"Yes!" she responded. "It must be broken because the time says 9:00 a.m., and it's pitch-black outside."

"Mom," I said, "in December in Stockholm, the sun does not rise until about 10:00 a.m. Then it will remain light for only four hours, after which time it will get dark again by 2:00 p.m."

She looked at me like I was crazy and remained puzzled over the matter. Then she said, "Just because you won the Nobel Prize does not mean you know everything."

As we ate our breakfast, our other guests came by, sat for a few moments, congratulated me, and thanked me for inviting them. Sharon and I rarely had a chance to be alone at breakfast, and we had to take advantage of rare moments to talk to one another. Often, the best we could manage was to smile at each other from a distance.

Soon after breakfast, the Laureates and their spouses were asked to attend an orientation where staff would explain the schedule and upcoming events for Nobel Week. We were told that this year's Nobel Prize in Medicine had attracted a great deal more attention from the public compared to previous years. The reason given was that the people closely relate to nitroglycerin, which Alfred Nobel had used to make his invention of dynamite over a century prior. They pointed out that, because of this, we might encounter large crowds of people outside the hotel, waiting to see us and asking for photos.

We each had several interviews with the local and international news media. During one interview, a newspaper reporter asked me if I was planning to give the money that accompanies the Nobel Prize to charity. The reporter told me that many Laureates do just that. I thought about it for a moment and then said, "Have you heard the phrase that charity begins at home? Well, I'm going to use the money to buy a home—a home in Beverly Hills." The reporter then asked me if I felt good about having figured out how an explosive like nitroglycerin could actually work as a beneficial heart drug.

My answer to the reporter was that my nitroglycerin research brings me as close to Alfred Nobel as does the Nobel Prize itself.

One highlight of the whole trip was when I was asked to make a guest appearance on a local TV show for children around twelve and thirteen years of age to explain the importance of nitric oxide in the body. The staff had constructed a large, lifelike cardboard model of an adult body, illustrating most major organs. I was asked to briefly explain the role of nitric oxide in each organ. I was pleased to see that the organs depicted did not project below the colon. Young children did not need to understand "all" of the actions of NO.

I was delighted when they were able to answer many of the questions I fired at them. It was clear that the educational system in Sweden prioritized teaching young kids about the Nobel Prize and what it means to society. The students understood that the Nobel Prize is awarded to major discoveries that benefit humankind. From my experience in the US, I haven't seen this kind of effort. Indeed, few children in the US know what the Nobel Prize is, and those who do believe that the prize is only for peace.

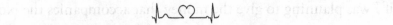

Los Angeles is sunny and warm nearly all year long, and many of us are spoiled because of that. Stockholm is situated much farther north, so daytime temperatures remained in the twenties, and the snow fell relentlessly day and night and never melted. The total accumulation after a week was over three feet. However, there was never any traffic congestion or walking problems because the city maintained all roads and sidewalks on a twenty-four-hour basis. The snow was a beautiful sight to behold.

Later that evening, after Sharon and I were separated for much of the day, we decided to go for a walk in the snow before retiring. The gentle sound of the snow falling was so relaxing, and the sight of the snowflakes in the lamppost-lighted sky was beautiful and romantic.

This walk in the snow was one of the few chances we'd had to be alone and take in what was happening around us. Looking across the harbor, we had a full view of the Grand Hotel, all lit up. The blowing snow created a beautiful halo effect around the lights of the hotel.

We talked about how both our moms were so delighted to be in Stockholm and were having a great time together. We felt sad that both our fathers had already passed away. My dad, in particular, would have been so proud of his son's accomplishments, and I would have loved to have seen his expression when I received the Nobel Prize. But, as my mom told me earlier that day, "Don't worry, son, your father is watching everything from up there."

As we headed back to the hotel, Sharon and I realized that we had been married for only fourteen months before the announcement of the prize. Moreover, we had dated for only six months prior to our marriage. She asked me if I still would have asked her out on a date had I already received the prize. I said, "What kind of a silly question is that? Of course, I would have!"

Then I asked Sharon if she would have accepted my dating request, as a Nobel Laureate, and she said she was not sure.

"Fair enough," I said. "But we don't have to worry about that now, do we?" I grabbed her arm, and we picked up our pace back to the hotel.

The following three days were filled with events such as the Nobel Laureate Lectures, luncheon events with ambassadors from various countries, concerts, photo sessions, and city tours. The lectures were divided up into the five categories of Nobel Prizes and were held at different times. The Nobel Lectures in Physiology or Medicine were held the morning of December 7. Robert Furchgott started things off, followed by Ferid Murad and then me, each of us giving a sixty-minute talk. I requested to go last because I've always enjoyed highlighting and summarizing the discoveries pertinent to nitric oxide. Moreover, I always display my sense of humor while lecturing, whereas Bob and Ferid are far too serious. With the audience having already sat for two hours, I was looking forward to making them laugh a bit.

The Nobel Prize Ceremony and Banquet are held on December 10, the anniversary of Alfred Nobel's death. The day of the Nobel Prize ceremony, I spent the morning in casual clothes at the Stockholm Concert Hall, where the Laureates underwent a thorough dress rehearsal to prepare for the real thing later that afternoon. This was the first time I can recall being trained how to march, turn corners, sit, stand, and bow in front of a king. Traditionally, the chairman of the institute awarding the prize announces the name of the Laureate, who then steps forward and walks across the stage to the king. The moderator then says something to the effect of, "Will [name of Laureate] please accept the Nobel Prize from the hands of His Majesty, the King?"

After receiving the prize, the Laureate first bows in front of the king and queen. He or she then turns gracefully to the back of the stage to face the members of the Nobel Foundation, and bows. Finally, the Laureate turns 180 degrees to face the audience, and bows, before returning to their seat. In my year, 1998, this was to be performed by nine Nobel Laureates.

The Nobel ceremony commenced at 4:00 p.m., but dressing for it began in the early afternoon with my struggle to figure out how to dress up in a white tie and tails. I found that solving a quadratic equation or balancing a complicated chemical reaction was far easier than this tuxedo project. With Sharon's help, I was able to put it all on without looking like a clown. I had to practice sitting and standing properly so I wouldn't step on my tails and pull myself to the ground by the neck.

Once dressed, I looked pretty good, and Sharon looked absolutely gorgeous in her new gown and shoes. She also put on a bit of makeup, which I had never seen her do except for our visit to the White House a few weeks earlier. We were ready to go.

We took the elevator down to the main lobby. When the doors opened, we saw dozens of people, all dressed up, wandering around. I immediately singled out Margarita, who was standing in the corner, waiting for us. She smiled ear to ear when she saw us all dressed up. She loved Sharon's gown and thought I looked "very intelligent" in my white tie and tails. Margarita also looked stunning in her beautiful gown and her hair all done up.

"How are you feeling?" she asked.

"Nervous, but ready to go!"

She explained that she would accompany Sharon and me in our limousine driven by Hans, whereas our family members and guests would be transported by large vans. She assured us that the families would be looked after and kept together for the remainder of the day and evening. I was relieved to learn that. After all the Laureates assembled, each couple was then escorted by their assigned attaché to their own limousine in preparation for all of us to depart from the Grand Hotel as one motorcade to the Stockholm Concert Hall.

As Sharon and I walked out the revolving doors at the hotel entrance, we saw crowds of people standing by to watch us exit. Everyone in the crowd was cheering and applauding as we walked by. This was something very special indeed, as it was completely unexpected. We entered our car and sat back, looking out the windows of the limousine at the impressive crowd and the motorcade flanked with police cars and motorcycles. Then, I saw the police escorts turn on their flashing lights, followed by the sound of sirens. The limousines started to inch forward. We were on our way to the Nobel Ceremony.

As the limousine slowly pulled away from the hotel, I could feel my heart pounding, and I grabbed on to Sharon's hand. All of a sudden, many of the key experiments from my lab flashed before my eyes. Then the afternoon spent at the Nobel Forum in Stockholm, where several Nobel committee members heard me speak, kept bouncing in and out of my head. I realized how fortunate I was that Mom was still alive and doing well so that she could witness all of this. She had lived a mostly sheltered life and had never experienced anything remotely similar to what was happening this day. Although Mom was in a separate vehicle with other members of our families, I knew that she must have been enjoying all of the commotion.

December 10 is a special date for the residents of Stockholm because of the celebration and awarding of the Nobel Prizes. Typically, they line the sidewalks adjacent to the streets all the way from the Grand Hotel to the Concert Hall. But in 1998, the crowd was much larger than in past years because of the connection between the Nobel Prize in Medicine, nitroglycerin, and Nobel himself.

As I looked out the windows, I saw that the crowds were at least ten rows deep, and everyone was covered in snow and cheering us on, as they waved Swedish flags and held up banners with the letter N, signifying Nobel. In one instance, I saw someone holding up a large banner inscribed with the word NITROGLYCERIN. The crowds were so large that, on occasion, the motorcade had to stop because of overflow into the street. As all of this was occurring, the snow kept falling as large, beautiful flakes, and I was daydreaming about what it might feel like when the king placed the Nobel Prize into my extended hands.

The limousines pulled up to the front entrance of the Concert Hall, one at a time. When it was our turn to exit the limousine, Margarita got out first and opened Sharon's door, while Hans opened mine. Margarita then explained that we were to walk on the red carpet all the way into the Hall. The red carpet looked beautiful as the thick snow accumulated on the surface. As I looked around, I could see that the large crowds had not dissipated one bit. In fact, the crowds had thickened, though they were kept on either side of the red carpet by barricades.

Margarita led us into the Concert Hall, where the Laureates were taken backstage. The nine of us chatted for about thirty minutes before the procession began. The music started, and we were told to get ready to march. The Royal Stockholm Philharmonic Orchestra, conducted by Sir Andrew Davis, began to play, and we were off. Mindful not to spoil the occasion by tripping over my tails, I paid careful attention to how and where I was walking.

The Concert Hall was filled with people and gorgeous flowers. As was tradition since the first Nobel Prize ceremony in 1901, the flower arrangements were brought in from San Remo, Italy, where Alfred Nobel passed away in 1896.

We marched to our designated seats onstage. The nine Nobel Laureates (Physics, Chemistry, Physiology or Medicine, Literature, and Economic Sciences) were seated on the left of center in the front row. The Nobel Laureates for the Peace Prize were conspicuous in their absence. The Peace Prize is awarded on precisely the same day and time but in nearby Oslo, Norway. This had been a tradition since Alfred Nobel made this request in his last will and testament. At that time, Norway was engaged in numerous peace initiatives, and Nobel wanted to recognize Norway for this accomplishment. The Nobel Laureates in Peace that year were John Hume and David Trimble.

Behind us were several rows of seats occupied by many special guests, including prior Nobel Laureates and distinguished people in the fields represented by the five categories of the Nobel Prizes. On the right side of center were several rows of seats filled by members of the five Nobel Prize Committees and members of the Nobel Assembly and Foundation. As I was walking to my seat in the front row, I glanced over to the second row and recognized Sir John Vane sitting right behind me. As we had to march to our seats in a professional manner, I subtly acknowledged his presence by smiling at him, and he smiled back.

The executive director of the Nobel Foundation, Michael Sohlman, made the opening remarks, first in Swedish, followed by English. The first to be called up were the three Laureates in Physics. As they were asked to stand, my heart rate jumped from about ninety to one hundred beats per minute, although I was still sitting down. My normal resting heart rate is below sixty. I knew my turn would soon come. Each of the Laureates was addressed individually and walked over to the king to accept the Nobel Prize medallion and diploma. Next came the Chemistry Laureate, who was introduced by the same man. Both the prizes in Physics and Chemistry are awarded by the Royal Swedish Academy of Sciences. As soon as he stood up, my heart rate climbed a bit higher because I knew we were next. Finally, it was our turn: the Nobel Laureates in Physiology or Medicine.

We were introduced, one at a time, by the chairman of the Nobel Assembly at the Karolinska Institute, Professor Sten Lindahl. First, he gave the audience a general description of why nitric oxide had been recognized. The first of us to meet the king and collect the Nobel Prize was Bob Furchgott, who looked very proud indeed. As he was returning to his seat, my heart felt like it was about to explode. It was my turn. Professor Lindahl called me by name and asked me to come forward to receive the Nobel Prize and diploma from the hands of His Majesty, the King. My heart thumped in my chest as I approached the king, who was standing and waiting for me in the center of the stage. The king was standing on a large symbol inscribed into the carpet—the letter N inside a large circle. Many thoughts raced through my mind in the few seconds it took to walk to center stage. My high school, college, and post-graduate training all flashed before my eyes as I approached the circle where the king was waiting to receive me. When I reached center stage, standing before the king, I glanced down at the carpet and thought to myself, *Look at this, the symbol of N with the O encircling it looks just like the symbol for nitric oxide, NO.* I looked back up and realized that *I was about to receive the Nobel Prize from the King of Sweden.*

After bowing to the king and queen and the distinguished people onstage, I turned to bow to the audience. During our morning rehearsal of the ceremony, we were taught the proper way to bow. The key was to look professional and reserved, holding back any emotional expression. I later found out that the local newspaper staff had a tradition of grading the posture and bowing technique of the Nobel Laureates and publishing the results in the next morning's newspaper. Never one to have a great poker face, my technique earned the ranking of dead last. Upon turning to face the audience, just prior to bowing, I displayed a big smile from ear to ear and wiggled both eyebrows a few times as if to say, "Wow, how do you like this? Isn't this great?"

After the remaining Laureates had received their prizes, the ceremony was brought to a close. The king and queen exited the stage. The Nobel Laureates and other people onstage remained so we could interact with one another. Our spouses were then escorted by staff onto the stage to join us. I spotted Sharon and gave her the biggest hug ever.

While onstage, I seized the opportunity to walk over to the three committee members who had attended my special lecture at the Nobel Forum in Stockholm a few months before the announcement of the Nobel Prize. I shook their hands and thanked them for their support. Then I singled out the committee member who had interrogated me after my Nobel Forum lecture. I told Professor Tomas Hökfelt that I would never forget our intense discussion but that I hadn't thought I'd be receiving the Nobel Prize in the same year. He was full of smiles and, in a soft-spoken voice, gave me his heartfelt congratulations.

Immediately thereafter, I walked over to Sir John Vane, who had been seated behind me in the second row during the ceremony. I told John, once again, how much he had inspired and motivated me to continue studying nitric oxide.

Our onstage celebration eventually ended, and Margarita appeared and escorted us to our limousine for the short ride to City Hall for the famous Nobel Banquet. By this time, I had developed quite an appetite. Margarita took Sharon and me to a room where we were gathered together to be a part of a procession that would march through a special elevated entrance and then down the staircase to our designated seats at the head of a long table of about ninety people. Seated in the center of the large table, but opposite one another, were King Carl Gustaf and Queen Silvia. Surrounding the head table on both sides were dozens of long tables placed perpendicular to the head table, each table seating about twenty-five people. Our family and invited guests were scattered among the side tables.

The banquet hosted about 1,200 people in total. During the evening, a multicourse meal was served by about 450 servers who had trained for several months prior to the banquet. They all marched in and out together to serve and clear each course in a procession of military-style perfection. The cuisine was excellent, as were the wines. The specially designed Nobel tableware was elegant and suited the occasion. In fact, the next morning, Sharon and I walked over to a special section of the NK department store to purchase one complete Nobel place setting, which we display in a lighted cabinet in our dining room at home.

Following the four-hour dinner, we marched out in predetermined order and were then guided by staff to the Gold Room, located upstairs. The Gold Room is a large hall used that evening as a ballroom, about 150 feet long and 100 feet wide, with ample room to accommodate well over a thousand people. The walls were lined with gold mosaic patterns created by the artist Einar Forseth on a proposal by the City Hall architect in 1918. The ball after the Nobel Banquet is always held in the Gold Room, and along the sides of the two longer walls, behind a series of brick pillars, sat displays of various memorabilia belonging to Alfred Nobel.

In addition, in several elegant glass cabinets, all nine Nobel Prizes and diplomas awarded in 1998 were on display for everyone to see. This evening was one to remember. Indeed, the entire day of December 10, 1998, was one of the most memorable of my life.

The Day After

Sharon and I returned to our room, totally exhausted. Nevertheless, I found it difficult to sleep after the events of the day, which seemed like several days rolled into one. We managed to wake up the next morning and have breakfast with the family, as we had done on each previous morning. The conversation was animated with lots of discussion about the Nobel Ceremony and Banquet.

My brother, Angelo, pointed out something he recognized onstage. "When each of the Laureates bowed in front of the audience, you were the only one who had a big smile on your face."

I explained that we were told in rehearsal not to smile or show any emotion when we bowed. "Obviously, I couldn't control myself."

Mom quickly cut in, "Why not?" she said. "You just got the Nobel Prize. Why shouldn't you smile?"

"Well, we were instructed to look formal because this was a very formal ceremony."

"That's so damn foolish!" Mom said. "I'm so glad you smiled!"

My mom was especially happy and repeatedly expressed how proud she was of her son.

"Well, you know Mom, I owe a lot to you and Dad for buying me that chemistry set when I was a kid. It enabled me to understand science much better and become a good scientist."

A concerned look formed on her face, "Yeah, I know that, but you didn't have to blow up the basement and fireplace to be a good scientist, did you?"

Angelo cut right in. "Mom, nobody else at the age of eleven or twelve could have achieved what Lou did. His perseverance was responsible for his success."

"Yeah, yeah, I know, but he's lucky to have any hands left after those explosions."

Knowing that no one could ever come out on top after a discussion with our mom, Angelo backed off.

Then, suddenly, I had a flashback. It had been about forty-five years since I'd built and set off my homemade bomb that destroyed one of the concrete pillars holding up the boardwalk in Long Beach, New York. I had never before confessed that to my mom, but I knew she suspected I might have had something to do with the explosion, which she had heard from many miles away.

I decided it was time to come clean.

"Mom, I know this is a long time ago, but do you remember a big explosion that occurred during the time I was making firecrackers and rocket fuel? The explosion was not at home but was several miles away."

"Yes, I remember. And I asked you if you had anything to do with it. Well, did you?"

I told her that I was the one who had set off that explosion and that I had set it off under the boardwalk and damaged part of it.

"I knew it all along," she said, "but I didn't say anything because I wasn't sure. It's a good thing you didn't injure or kill anyone!" Mom pointed her finger right at me and, looking serious, said, "That was no fourth of July firecracker; that was a real bomb. You know, Nobel and you had something in common. Are you sure you weren't trying to make a stick of dynamite? If you blew up the boardwalk, then you made dynamite!"

Everyone at the table laughed.

"Are you sure you just won the Nobel Prize? What other Nobel Prize winners blew up a boardwalk?"

Once again, everyone erupted in laughter, including Mom this time.

After breakfast, Margarita came to fetch Sharon and me and remind us that we had to get ready to go to the Nobel Foundation to collect my Nobel Prize medal and diploma and to take care of important paperwork. The next morning, we got dressed in our usual business attire, and the limo took us to the Nobel Foundation, just two miles from the hotel, where we were introduced to the foundation's executive director, Michael Sohlman. He and Margarita escorted us to a special room upstairs, and the first matter of business was to hand over the Nobel Prize and the special diploma or certificate. Finally, I got the chance to touch and feel and study the Nobel Prize. *How elegant*, I thought.

The Nobel Prize medallion for Physiology or Medicine is also referred to as the medal of the Nobel Assembly at the Karolinska Institute because this particular prize is awarded by the Nobel Assembly at the Karolinska. The twenty-four-karat gold medal is about 2.5 inches in diameter, and the front side has an etching of the face of Alfred Nobel. The back side of the medal has a beautiful etching representing the Genius of Medicine holding an open book in her lap, collecting the water pouring out from a rock to quench a sick girl's thirst. The inscription around the edge of the medal reads *Inventas vitam iuvat excoluisse per artes*, which loosely translates as, "And they who bettered life on Earth by their newly found mastery." (Word for word: inventions enhance life which is beautified through art.) The words are taken from Vergilius Aeneid, the sixth song, verse 663: "*Lo, God-loved poets, men who spake things worthy Phoebus' heart; and they who bettered life on earth by new-found mastery."*

Finally, at the bottom, just under the etching, is my name, L. J. Ignarro, and the year 1998 written in Roman numerals as MCMXCVIII.

The next order of business was also the highlight of the day, perhaps the entire week, when I was asked to add my signature to a special book that contained the signatures of all Nobel Laureates who had come before me.

Before signing my name, Michael Sohlman asked that I carefully turn through the pages of signatures, beginning with the first one in 1901. There was the signature of Wilhelm Conrad Röntgen, who was awarded the first Nobel Prize in Physics, for his discovery of X-ray radiation. I turned only a few pages and saw the signature of Marie Curie, who was awarded the Nobel Prize in Physics in 1903 for her discovery of radioactivity. Moving along, I saw the signature of Guglielmo Marconi, who was awarded the Physics Prize in 1909 for the invention of wireless telegraphy. I got more excited when I saw Marie Curie's signature for the second time, this one in 1911 in Chemistry, for her discovery of several new radioactive elements.

The moment my eyes ran across the signature of Albert Einstein, who was awarded the Nobel Prize in Physics in 1922, I paused and immediately became teary-eyed because of the significance of this scientist. I said out loud, "How is it possible that I am about to add my signature to a book that contains the signature of Albert Einstein?"

Then I recognized the signatures of Frederick Grant Banting in 1923 for the discovery of insulin, and Alexander Fleming in 1945 for the discovery of penicillin and its curative effect in various infectious diseases. It was truly unbelievable to see the signatures of so many individuals who made world-changing discoveries.

As I turned the pages, I became excited at the prospect of seeing the signatures of several Nobel Laureates who had influenced my life and career. These included Linus Pauling (1954, Chemistry), Julius Axelrod (1970, Medicine), Christian de Duve (1974, Medicine), Andrew Schally (1977, Medicine), John Vane (1982, Medicine), and Paul Boyer (1997, Chemistry).

What a humbling experience!

"Okay," I said out loud. "Now it's my turn!"

I was given a special pen, a quill pen, to use. I'd never seen such a pen before. Essentially, it was a feather about ten inches in length. Once the tip was dipped into the ink well, the ink was absorbed up into the stem of the feather and flowed evenly to the paper by capillary action. I didn't think I would be able to use this thing without making a mess of the signature page in the book. But I practiced a few times on scrap paper, and it worked amazingly well.

After my hand stopped trembling, I took a deep breath and added my signature to this special Nobel book. So many thoughts went through my mind in the second or two it took to sign my name. The most prominent thought was my dad, who never understood what science was but worked with me and supported me when I was a child. I so wished that he could be alive to witness this special day in my life.

Next, it was about time for me to dress up in my favorite costume once again—the white tie and tails. In a couple of hours, we would be off to the castle to have dinner with King Carl Gustaf and Queen Silvia. After having experienced the feeling of adding my signature to such a special book, I figured that another evening out to dinner would be anticlimactic. I was wrong.

About thirty people were in attendance. These included King Carl Gustaf and Queen Silvia, the nine Nobel Laureates and their spouses, the director of the foundation together with other key members and their spouses, and several members of the royal family, including Princess Lilian. The evening was more relaxed than the celebration the night of the ceremony. Each guest had ample opportunity to chat with the royalty as well as with one another. Following the exquisite dinner, we all were escorted to visit several beautiful rooms within the castle, where we could take photographs and enjoy some brandy and smoking, if that was your pleasure, as well as converse with the king and queen. Both the king and queen took the group of us for a tour through some rooms in the castle, and each took turns explaining the significance of each room and its contents.

In talking with Queen Silvia, we learned that she was not Swedish but rather half-German and half-Brazilian. King Carl Gustaf, of course, was Swedish, and both were delightful conversationalists. What struck many of us about the king was his uncanny ability to hold a brandy glass and a burning cigar in one hand, while walking around and shaking hands with his free hand, never spilling a drop of brandy. I couldn't even manage to hold just the brandy glass and shake hands without spillage.

Once again, Sharon and I were exhausted when we returned to our hotel room. After taking one more glimpse of my Nobel Prize, we packed our suitcases for the trip home the next morning.

We were in a deep sleep when we were suddenly awakened at 6:00 a.m. by candlelight and music at the foot of our bed. After clearing our eyes, we saw six golden-haired young ladies with lighted candles on their heads, singing carols at our bedside. Then we heard them singing "Santa Lucia." We later learned that this was based on Lucia Day, when Swedes brighten up the darkest period of the year with celebrations embracing a Roman Catholic martyr and a light festival which pre-dates Christianity. Though Lucia Day was not until December 21 (the shortest day of the year), they always hold a preview of their traditions on December 12 for the Nobel Laureates at the end of Nobel Week.

This unforgettable event was followed by the ladies serving us breakfast in bed. The whole thing was like a dream. I actually thought that I had died and gone to heaven. But I snapped out of it, realizing that we had to wash up and get ready for our flight back home.

Margarita greeted us in the lobby and escorted us to our limousine, bound for the airport. Just as when we had arrived eight days earlier, it was snowing.

Upon arrival at LAX, we collected our luggage and walked over to the long-term parking lot where I had left my car for over a week. There was no Margarita to escort us to the car, but we located it, nevertheless. When we reached the car, out of habit, I climbed into the rear seat, waiting for my driver, Hans, to take us home.

"Very funny!" Sharon said. "Come on, let's go."

PART V:
Post-Nobel and New Findings

"Logic will get you from point A to point B, but imagination will take you everywhere."
— Albert Einstein

Chapter 17:
A Centennial to Remember

The Nobel Prize changed my life completely. Research funding opportunities improved dramatically, even though I did not need any more funds to adequately execute my research program. The number of student applications to my research program increased tenfold, but I did not take advantage of this because I've always maintained a relatively small group, consisting of no more than a dozen people at any one time.

An opportunity arose at UCLA to develop a cardiovascular research institute. Had I seized upon it, I would have named it the Center for Nitric Oxide Research (CNOR). But I was uncertain if I wanted to assume such responsibility. At the same time, I was receiving and accepting many speaking invitations worldwide. This had never happened to me, and I was enjoying the opportunity to travel all around the world.

Other institutions began to court me. A nearby university, Cedars-Sinai, also offered to build me a research institute with a productive nitric oxide research program. Our big rival, USC, was keen to recruit me and my entire research program. But none could entice me to leave UCLA.

My decisions turned out just fine. I continued to enjoy my new lifestyle of fame, travel, and expanded opportunities. For example, I was asked to consider chairmanship positions at several medical schools throughout the country. I was overwhelmed and flattered by all of this. Never before had I received this much attention. However, in the end, I concluded that I was happy with my small research group at UCLA and chose to remain right where I was.

Several exciting opportunities arose during my tenure at UCLA. In 1999, while traveling in Italy to give a lecture on my work, Dr. Alessandro Casini, a high-level director at the Menarini Pharmaceutical Company located in Florence, approached me with a plan to fund my research program if I would agree to examine the mechanism of action of one of their cardiovascular drugs used clinically to lower high blood pressure.

Since he felt that NO might be involved, and because such collaboration would require frequent trips to Florence to discuss the data, I quickly accepted his kind invitation. We are still collaborating to this very day. Sharon and I have been to Italy dozens of times on invitation by Menarini. We've attended so many conferences on the Isle of Capri that we seriously considered buying a small home there, with a spectacular view of the Mediterranean Sea and the coast of Italy. But logistics posed a serious problem for us. That is, we were not certain if we could manage foreign properties while residing in LA. The nature of my profession, and Sharon's as an anesthesiologist, demanded that we spend the great majority of our time in LA. And what would we do with our two beautiful golden retrievers?

In the spring of 2001, I received a letter of invitation from the Nobel Foundation, informing me that the Nobel Foundation planned to hold its first centennial celebration of the Nobel Prize.

Spectacular, I thought. The letter went on to state that all living Nobel Laureates and their spouses were invited to participate, at the expense of the Nobel Foundation. The estimated number of Nobel Laureates to attend was approximately 155 and would include Laureates in all categories except Peace. The Nobel Peace Prize centennial was to be held simultaneously, but in Oslo, Norway.

Sharon and I quickly accepted the invitation.

I was looking forward to seeing the many Laureates I already knew. In particular, I was anxious to renew my acquaintances with Chris de Duve, Julie Axelrod, Andrew Schally, Sir John Vane, Paul Greengard, and Paul Boyer. Each of these scientists had been instrumental in setting a path for the forward development of my research career. But I was not certain whether any of them planned to attend.

I was lucky to have interacted with these individuals, none of whom had yet received their prize during our earlier encounters. My great plan was to find all six individuals early during Nobel

Week and request that we all get together so that I could explain to the group how each one had helped me during my research career.

Five months passed quickly, and before we knew it, we were on our way to Stockholm for this special celebration. While resting in the airport VIP lounge during one of our layovers, a gentleman walked in and sat in the opposite corner of the lounge. I did not recognize him, but he was conspicuous by the small, round, brass lapel pin on his suit jacket. The lapel pin was unmistakably a Nobel pin, given to every Nobel Laureate during the first day of Nobel Week. The face of the pin is identical to the front side of the Nobel Prize medallion.

I was wearing the same pin on my blazer, which also caught the gentleman's attention. He saw me looking at him and quickly turned away, as if to avoid me. Being the extrovert that I am, I walked over to introduce myself. "I am Lou Ignarro, and my lucky day was three years ago, in 1998."

"What field are you in?" he asked.

"I am a physiologist/pharmacologist, and my Prize was in Physiology or Medicine. How about you?"

"My name is John Nash," he answered, without making eye contact. "I was awarded the Nobel Prize in Economic Sciences in 1994."

I noticed right away he was rather shy and did not appear to enjoy much interaction. Therefore, I said, "It was nice to meet you, Dr. Nash. Have a safe continuing journey, and I'll see you soon in Stockholm."

He did not respond, so I walked away.

While Stockholm was cold, unlike 1998, there was no snow. As before, we were greeted at the airport and driven to the Grand Hotel, where we stayed for about six days. However, we had no private attaché or limousine driver. We had no Margarita or Hans to escort us. Still, everything was organized quite well. We spent the afternoon walking around Stockholm, enjoyed a light dinner, and retired early for the evening.

On awakening the following morning, we dressed in our gym clothes and went to the hotel fitness center for a good workout. As we entered the gym, I noticed a gentleman using a stationary bicycle. Oddly, he was wearing a suit and tie while riding the bike. My curiosity ignited, I slowly walked over to him. Then, in a flash, I recognized him.

"Julie! It's Lou Ignarro. How the hell are you? Long time no see!" Julius Axelrod was one of the people I had most hoped would attend the centennial.

He turned around and recognized me right away.

"Hello, Lou! It's so nice to see you again, after all these years." I then introduced him to Sharon, who was standing right by me.

"Julie, do you always work out in your suit?" I asked.

"I just wanted to move my legs a bit and get the blood flowing before sitting down for breakfast."

"Great idea," I said. "Sharon and I are going to work out as well before we go to breakfast. See you later."

Our second day in Stockholm promised to be special. The Foundation organized an event at City Hall for all attending Nobel Laureates and their spouses. The large hall was conducive to walking around and mingling. By the time everyone had walked into the hall, I was surrounded by over 150 Nobel Laureates! *Truly amazing*, I thought. *Who would have ever thought that I would be standing in the same room with so many Nobel Prize winners?* It was mind-boggling, indeed. To this day, I can't get over it.

As we entered the large hall, each of us was given a booklet that contained the photographs and names of the Nobel Laureates in attendance, 154 in all. As Sharon and I continued to walk through the hall, I kept reaching for the delicious hors d'oeuvres that were offered to us. I could not devour enough of the Swedish meatballs (Svenska Köttbullar) and cheese marinated in brandy with vanilla (Vaniljmarinerad Västerbottensost). Even my Marinella silk tie from Naples, Italy, got a good taste of the Swedish meatballs. As I was attempting to clean my tie, Dr. Andrew Schally and his wife came by. Andrew Schally had been at the VA Hospital in New Orleans while I was next door at Tulane Medical Center.

When I first met Schally about twenty-four years prior, he had not been very talkative, at least not with me. But this time, things were different. He recognized me first and said hello and then introduced Sharon and me to his wife, Ana Maria, at which time I introduced Sharon. Schally and I reminisced about the three-story-high chromatography columns he had constructed and used to separate and purify various peptides.

In the distance, I saw Professor Al Gilman and his wife, Kathryn, from Dallas. I grabbed Sharon's hand and scooted over to greet them, pausing on the way for more Swedish meatballs. I had known Al since 1970, during my early days working on cyclic GMP. Al was chairman of the Department of Pharmacology at Southwestern Medical School in Dallas, and he was an internationally renowned pharmacologist, known for his research on cell signaling, involving the action of cyclic AMP. Since cyclic GMP and cyclic AMP were distinct cyclic nucleotides but related due to their function as signaling molecules, Al and I had attended and participated in dozens of the same scientific conferences over a twenty-year period during the 1970s and '80s. Al Gilman had been awarded the Nobel Prize in Physiology or Medicine in 1994 for his discovery of G-proteins, which allow chemical signals to be transmitted to the interior of cells to elevate cyclic AMP levels.

As Sharon and I were finishing up with Al and Kathryn, someone tapped me on the shoulder. I turned around, and my face broke out in a big smile. It was Professor Christian de Duve from Rockefeller University in New York City. Chris de Duve was one of the most inspiring persons I had met early in my career as a pharmacologist. I was delighted that Chris recognized me. It had been about twenty-eight years since we had last seen each other in person. We exchanged hellos, and I commented on how well he looked.

"Well, you know that I am eighty-four years of age. I feel okay but moving around more slowly than before."

"You still look great," I added.

I asked him if Professor George Palade was also present at the centennial. Palade was a Romanian cell biologist who had shared the 1974 Nobel Prize in Physiology or Medicine with de Duve. Palade revolutionized the way we think about the nature and function of intracellular components of the cell and is still considered the most influential cell biologist ever.

Chris told me that George could not make it to the centennial because of his failing health.

As Sharon and I continued to walk through the distinguished crowd, I saw Paul Greengard directly in front of me. He was standing with a woman, who I suspected was his wife. He turned slightly and saw us approaching.

After exchanging pleasantries and introducing our wives, Paul and I stepped back about thirty years and recalled our discussions about cyclic GMP.

"Lou, I noted many years ago that you followed my lead and got the hell out of the drug industry."

"Yes, I certainly did just that. Although I was productive in drug discovery, my return to academia was incredibly rewarding in that I had the freedom to do any kind of research my heart desired."

"Yes, indeed! And I also noted that you stuck with cyclic GMP, just as I suggested you do. And now look what happened. You got the Nobel Prize!"

"Paul, there's no question in my mind that you steered me in the right direction. Thank you."

"When you received the Nobel just a few years back, you know what I told everyone around me?"

"No, what did you say?"

"I said, 'I know that guy. He's Lou Ignarro. We've known each other from the days of Geigy Pharmaceuticals in New York. I told him to quit the drug industry and go back to academics, and he did just that!'"

The next person I looked forward to seeing was Paul Boyer, who taught me enzymology and biochemistry at the University of Minnesota during my graduate studies. However, I learned from Sir John Walker, who shared the Nobel Prize in Chemistry with Paul in 1997, that Paul and his wife, Lydia, were not able to make it to Stockholm because Paul had the flu.

Then Sharon told me that she was going to walk around the entire hall and ask every Nobel Laureate to sign her Nobel Jubilee Photo Directory. I promptly told her not to do that because it would be considered impolite. However, one of the Physics Laureates in my year of 1998, Professor Horst Störmer, overheard our exchange and told me that Sharon's idea was a fabulous one. Without delay, he grabbed her hand and escorted her all around the hall for at least an hour.

While Horst and Sharon were gallivanting around, I approached each of the Laureates who I felt had positively impacted my professional career and asked them if we could all gather for a brief moment, a reunion of sorts, so that I could say a few words of thanks. I managed to assemble a group consisting of Julie Axelrod, Paul Greengard, Chris de Duve, Andrew Schally, and John Vane.

As we were gathered together, I said, "Thanks for agreeing to meet briefly. I want to begin my remarks with a toast."

I called over one of the waiters and asked him to kindly bring us six glasses of champagne. In a few moments, he was back with six glasses and a bottle of Dom Perignon, and he poured each of us a glass. I asked for everyone's attention and began to speak.

"This small gathering means a great deal to me because each of you played an instrumental role in setting the path for my success as a scientist, and I wanted each of you to understand why. Moreover, I've dreamed about organizing this reunion for several months prior to the centennial.

"I cannot express in words what it means to me to be standing here in Stockholm as a Nobel Laureate before the five Nobel Laureates who changed my life."

A loud sound of cheers followed as we took a sip of our Dom Perignon. I was about to explain how each of them influenced my basic research career when Julie cut in.

"But, Lou, how did I contribute to your success?"

"Julie, don't you remember? You opened your laboratory at the NIH to me despite the fact that I was a postdoctoral fellow in a different lab."

"Yes, I do recall you coming to my lab frequently," he said with a big grin. "But we were not working on nitric oxide or cyclic GMP at the time. Neither molecule had been discovered yet. So, what did you find appealing about my lab?"

I continued, "Because your systematic approach to pharmacology rubbed off on me. Moreover, and more importantly, I was struck by your attitude about opening up your laboratory to me because I wanted to learn more pharmacology. You encouraged me to work with your postdoctoral fellows whenever I had the time to come to your lab."

Chris de Duve added, "Lou, that seems to be a habit of yours. You would frequently visit my lab at Rockefeller University as well."

"Yes, that's true," I said. "I guess I have an insatiable capacity for knowledge, and I certainly learned a great deal from both of you."

Then, as I was about to continue speaking, Paul Greengard cut in.

"I know exactly why I had a positive influence on your career. I just told you that earlier this afternoon. Should I repeat it in front of this group?"

"Yes, of course," I said.

"It was twofold. First, I introduced Lou to cyclic GMP, from which I made my career. Second, I strongly encouraged Lou to leave the drug industry to embark on an unrestricted academic career in basic research."

"So that's why you left Geigy Pharmaceuticals," Chris added.

"It was a risky but damn good move," John commented.

"Moreover," Paul added, "I, too, had worked in the drug industry but made the move to academia, which provided the freedom to engage in basic research of my choosing and not what the company wanted me to do."

Chris jumped in. "Lou," he said, "I could not have influenced your discoveries on NO because I had never worked with this molecule. Perhaps I helped you better understand the inflammatory process during your visits to my cell biology lab in New York City? Your work at Geigy Pharmaceuticals resulted in the development and marketing of diclofenac (Voltaren, a novel anti-inflammatory drug for arthritis. And I was especially pleased because you discovered this compound by finding that it stabilized lysosomes and prevented inflammation by this mechanism."

That was news to the other gentlemen in the discussion, who broke out with loud cheers. It was time for more Dom Perignon.

Next, Andrew Schally stepped up to the plate and told the others how I had taken advantage of his methodology and applied his basic principles to purify enzyme proteins we were working with in our laboratory. He went on to explain the uniqueness of his long chromatographic columns, which I knew he was proud of.

"Did you people know that I constructed the longest chromatography columns in the world to purify peptides such as TRH, or thyrotropin-releasing hormone, from the hypothalamus?"

"Just how long were they?" asked John.

I could hear faint snickering among the group, but I don't think Andrew caught on. Andrew answered, "One column was twenty-five feet long, and another was twenty-one feet long."

What followed were some "wow" and an "oh my God" comments from the group. Andrew explained that such column length was necessary to achieve complete separation of the peptides from small proteins.

Then Paul Greengard asked me if I had worked with Andrew on this project.

Before I could answer, Andrew said, "No, my own laboratory accomplished that without any outside help."

Then he continued, "Lou, I recall that about twenty-five years ago, you came over to the Veterans Administration Hospital on the day of the announcement of my Nobel Prize. That was very nice of you."

More cheers and Dom Perignon followed.

Finally, John Vane entered into the group discussion with his usual forceful voice. "I know exactly how I was helpful to you, Lou. When I met you in New Orleans many years ago, I told you to pursue your studies on nitric oxide. And that was before you suspected that EDRF was NO. Then, a few years after that, if I recall correctly, you telephoned me in London to tell me you believed that EDRF was indeed NO."

"Yes, I asked you for your opinion regarding my hypothesis," I added.

"Yes, you did, and what did I tell you? I told you that you needed to test and prove your hypothesis. Furthermore, I told you not to let anything stand in your way of achieving that singularly important goal."

John knew all about the experiments we had conducted to demonstrate that EDRF was NO, but the others in the group did not. So, John explained the details to the group. I didn't have to say a thing. But I did shout out, "Cheers! Let's drink to that!" At about this time, one thing was certain: I was feeling the effects of the Dom Perignon!

Just as we were wrapping up our mini-celebration, Sharon and Horst came by, waving her Nobel booklet with signatures. After I introduced Horst to the five gentlemen in the group, he asked each of them to kindly sign their names next to their respective photos. They all agreed, and Sharon was delighted. Paul Greengard flipped through the pages and said, "Sharon, you could sell this booklet for thousands of dollars."

"Oh no," she said. "This treasure will go into our Nobel Room at home."

I thanked each of them for spending time with me at the centennial, and I became teary-eyed when we parted company, just as I am now, while writing this.

Sharon told me that she had gathered nearly a hundred signatures. Everyone she asked had been delighted to sign their name next to their photo. And to think that I had told her not to do this!

The special event ended, and we were driven back to the Grand Hotel.

As we entered the hotel lobby, we ran into Professor James Watson, whom I had not formally met before. Jim Watson shared the 1962 Nobel Prize in Physiology or Medicine with Francis Crick and Maurice Wilkins for their discovery of the double helix structure of the DNA molecule. Many prominent biologists and Nobel Laureates have described this discovery as the most significant and important biomedical discovery of the twentieth century, as it set the stage for fifty years of world-changing discoveries that followed.

I introduced myself and Sharon too. We all shook hands, and I promptly acknowledged him by saying, "Congratulations for your earth-shattering discovery of the double helix structure of DNA."

Without delay, he accepted my congratulations and proceeded to tell me how important his discovery was to the world.

Although I kept saying, "Yes sir, I know that," he kept going on and on.

Then, suddenly, he stopped and said, "What did you say your name was again?"

"Lou Ignarro. I was awarded the prize in 1998, just three years ago."

"So, tell me, why did you win the prize?"

I told him, "For the discovery of nitric oxide as a signaling molecule in the cardiovascular system."

Watson then asked me to explain what nitric oxide does in the cardiovascular system, and I told him, briefly.

"So, tell me, why was such a discovery so important to warrant a Nobel?"

Not knowing exactly how to answer his seemingly disparaging and contemptuous question, I answered, "Nitric oxide causes penile erections, and I am known as the Father of Viagra."

My answer perked him up. "Now, that *is* important!"

Chapter 18:

Back in Los Angeles

U pon returning home to Beverly Hills, I was confronted with a large pile of mail. This was always the price to pay for being away from home for a week or more. But before attacking the pile, I decided to relax for a few more days and reminisce about my recent experience in Stockholm. How many people have had the opportunity in their careers to mingle with over 150 Nobel Laureates for several days? I spent hours at a time just looking back on my interactions with so many Laureates, especially those who were instrumental in creating the road that led me to Stockholm. Sharon could see that I was daydreaming for days, and it was obvious to her that it was about our recent experiences in Stockholm.

She followed up with, "You enjoyed that, didn't you?"

"What a truly amazing week, don't you think?"

"You should be so proud," she said. "And I'm so proud of you!"

Then, while watching TV that evening, I saw that a special film was about to be released called *A Beautiful Mind* starring

Russell Crowe. It was a biopic of John Nash, whom I had met two weeks earlier on the way to Stockholm. Sharon and I went to see the film and found it quite moving. Although my only acquaintance with Professor Nash was brief, I was able to discern some similarities between him in person and the character played in the film. He was most definitely shy and preferred to be alone rather than making conversation in groups. During any conversation, he would not look straight at the person he was speaking to. His answers to any questions were no more than a few words, and he never raised any questions himself.

After a few days, I couldn't put it off anymore. It was time to buckle down and look at what the mail had in store for me. As I sifted through the pile, I noticed correspondence from pharmaceutical and cosmetic companies, where I was being asked to join their Scientific Advisory Board, Board of Directors, or collaborate with them on product development. One exciting opportunity was from the Lancôme division of L'Oréal in Paris, France. The cosmetics company had asked me to collaborate with them to develop novel skin cream products. At first, I wondered why the company would want me to work with them, as I knew absolutely nothing about cosmetics. Then, they explained that they wanted advice on two different kinds of cosmetic creams. One was for eliminating blemishes and discolorations while making the skin a bit whiter in color. The other product was for enhancing the tanning of the skin without adding artificial chemicals that would make the skin look yellow. Both of these effects, though opposite in nature, involved nitric oxide.

I accepted the invitation to collaborate with Lancôme, and our interaction turned out to be well worth my while. The frequent visits to Paris and New York City enhanced the overall experience. One of their new skin cream products was based on quenching or blocking the actions of nitric oxide in the dermal layers of the skin. Since NO causes the skin to darken, quenching the effects of NO in the skin would lighten the color of the outer skin layers. This product (Absolue Revitalizing and Brightening Soft Cream) became a big success in Asian countries like Japan, where women prefer a whiter color to their skin.

I also accepted an invitation to serve on the board of directors of a Los Angeles-based startup pharmaceutical company, CytRx. This turned out to be a rewarding experience, not only in helping to develop drugs and getting them to market, but also learning much more about business practices in general, a subject in which I'd received no previous training. To this day, I am still on the board of directors at CytRx.

While all of this was going on, I also began collaborating with scientific investigators in foreign countries, including Italy, Japan, South Korea, and Saudi Arabia. I was a visiting professor for several years at Nagoya University in Japan, Konkuk University in Seoul, South Korea, and King Saud College of Medicine in Riyadh, Saudi Arabia. These collaborations were truly escapades, and I enjoyed each one.

My experiences in Japan were highly rewarding because I established a close collaborative arrangement with Professor Toshio Hayashi, who had been a postdoctoral fellow in my lab at UCLA back in 1992, before he became a professor of gerontology at Nagoya University School of Medicine. We enjoyed the opportunity to join forces again. On every one of my dozens of visits over a five-year period, he would greet me on arrival at the Nagoya airport and take me back to the airport on my departure for home.

He knew that I was a big fan of sushi, and we never missed a sushi dinner together in Nagoya. Indeed, on many occasions, Toshio would take me on the bullet train (Shinkansen) to Tokyo for exquisite sushi, the finest in the world. The collaboration with Toshio has lasted for many years since my first visit to Nagoya, and we have published many important studies together dealing with nitric oxide and its role in a healthy lifestyle.

My collaborative program in Naples, Italy, did not involve any formal university appointment. I met a physician-scientist, Professor Claudio Napoli, while attending a planning meeting with the Menarini pharmaceutical company in Capri. Claudio and I became good collaborators and close friends. In addition, I continued my working relationship with Professor Giuseppe (Pippo) Cirino, also in Naples. These friendships resulted in my visiting Naples several times each year, which was such a treat because it was my dad's birthplace.

However, all of these extracurricular activities began to take a toll on my capacity to run an effective and productive research program at UCLA. Accordingly, about three years post-Nobel Prize, I made one of the most difficult decisions of my career. I decided to stop conducting basic academic research at UCLA.

Nevertheless, this is what I wanted to do with the remainder of my life. The Nobel Prize spoiled me rotten because it opened up so many other exciting opportunities that would never have been available to me without such recognition. I decided to stop raising new funds for my laboratory, allowing the three or four years of remaining funds to become depleted. I stopped recruiting new graduate students and postdoctoral fellows. In addition, I stopped my teaching activities, which was another difficult decision for me.

Part of my reason to downsize was another exciting business opportunity that arose in 2003. Stemming from my collaborative efforts on NO production from L-arginine, I had an idea for a nutritional supplement product that would increase the production and action of nitric oxide in our blood vessels. Such a product would consist of a mixture of L-arginine, L-citrulline, and several antioxidants that could be added to water or juice for consumption. This idea was based on my original basic research in collaboration with my colleagues in Naples and Nagoya. And so, I started up my own company to design and develop such heart-healthy products. I soon discovered, however, that a great deal of funds were required to achieve my goals. Fortunately, I was introduced to the executive management team at Herbalife Nutrition, which was interested in doing business with me. We established a productive and long-lasting relationship to this very day.

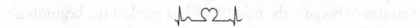

A Day on the Hill

In early 2000, I received a telephone call from an official at the National Institutes of Health (NIH) in Bethesda, Maryland. He asked me if I would consider being appointed to a small team of scientists charged with the task of meeting before the House Subcommittee on Health to argue why the NIH budget should be increased. This House Subcommittee is a Standing Committee of the House Energy and Commerce Committee that has general jurisdiction over bills and resolutions relating to numerous health-related organizations and institutions, including the NIH. The NIH provides the largest percentage of financial support for university-based biotech research. The NIH annual budget in 1998 was approximately $13 billion, which was insufficient to support the rapidly growing number of excellent research proposals submitted to the NIH for funding. This deficiency led to an outcry from the biomedical research community for an increase in the NIH budget. I was told that my name, in particular, had come up for two reasons. First, the NIH had supported my basic research budget for the previous thirty-eight years. Second, I was a recent Nobel Laureate in Physiology or Medicine, and such an accolade had resulted from my basic research, largely funded by the NIH.

I saw this as an excellent opportunity for me to help tens of thousands of American biomedical scientists receive competitive funding to support their individual basic research projects. It also was timely because the mid-1990s had marked the beginning of difficult times for investigators to receive adequate funding to support their programs. More and more young scientists were coming on to the scene and competing for funds at the fixed NIH annual budget, between $10 billion and $13 billion. Young scientists were finding it difficult, if not impossible, to get started. Moreover, veteran scientists were running into great difficulty keeping their long-established laboratories afloat. Only one thing could possibly save both young and established investigators, and that was a substantial increase in the NIH budget. And so, off I went to Washington, DC, to play politics.

Our small team consisted of about six prominent, internationally well-recognized scientists in the biomedical sciences. We each started off by giving a five- to ten-minute talk about why we felt the NIH annual budget should be increased. This was followed by questions from the six-member House Subcommittee on Health. After breaking for lunch, we resumed our discussions.

The questions from the Representatives of the House were direct and forceful. They demanded to understand exactly why the government should appropriate billions of dollars more to enable more biomedical research. As a team, we argued that the health of American citizens is more important than anything else the government had to accomplish with its budget. One would have thought that such an argument would be sufficient, but the subcommittee kept going on and on about other important matters that also necessitated more funding.

The hour was getting late, we were getting frustrated, and my colleagues were ready to quit. Then, I suddenly perked up as if I had just received an intravenous shot of espresso. I quickly put my thoughts together and commenced to deliver my final case for more funding.

I explained, in layman's terms with a twist of politics, what my contributions to medicine were that had resulted in my Nobel Prize. I then got personal and told them of my family.

"My mom and dad were immigrants from Italy and never attended schooling of any kind. And despite that handicap, I was able to climb to the top of my profession." I ended my comments by saying, "Distinguished members of the House Subcommittee, only in America can the son of an immigrant carpenter win the Nobel Prize."

The room went silent for nearly thirty seconds. Finally, the representatives thanked us for speaking, and the meeting was adjourned.

Although the meeting in Washington, DC, left us with doubt as to its outcome, I felt good about myself as I took my flight back to LA. Months went by, and then we were informed that the House Subcommittee had approved our request to increase the NIH budget. This was fantastic news, *but by how much*, I wondered.

A few weeks later, we learned that President Bill Clinton had supported the subcommittee's request to nearly double the NIH annual budget over the next four years. We had not expected that kind of a budget increase, if any increase at all. President Clinton's term ended in January of 2001, and George W. Bush took over as president. One year later, in 2002, President Bush followed through with a proposal, as recommended by the House

Subcommittee, to increase the NIH budget from $13 billion to $27 billion. As the next few years went by, many more young investigators received funding, and the more established scientists were able to hang on to their labs for at least a while longer.

Chapter 19:
The Nobel Prize Changed My Life

T he Nobel Prize opened up countless speaking opportunities for Bob Furchgott, Ferid Murad, and me to share about our research findings at conferences and institutions. We each received many individual invitations to travel globally and speak about our discoveries. But I took a somewhat different approach. I did not want to focus only on my research accomplishments. Anyone interested in the details could easily read the literature. I held a steadfast belief that nitric oxide had a bright future ahead, with many new discoveries still to be made, and I wanted to encourage investigators to expand the horizons of this magic molecule. So, I devoted most of my time telling audiences of scientists what I believed was the necessary basic research to determine how NO was instrumental in promoting and maintaining health as we age. My lectures at many conferences focused on a hypothesis that I had developed over many years that the continuous production of nitric oxide by vascular endothelial cells could turn out to be critical to the maintenance of cardiovascular health and longevity, and I argued that this hypothesis needed to be tested critically. I asked for any interested scientists to consider this area of basic research.

My goal was to entice and motivate other investigators to study whether there was any relationship between diet and NO production. Moreover, I argued that it was imperative to determine the impact of physical activity on the production of NO. I explained my belief that continuous NO production was closely linked to a healthy diet and moderate physical activity and that this hypothesis needed to be widely tested. My approach paid off because many investigators, including small startup biotech companies and other organizations, launched their own studies on the physiological roles of NO in health and disease.

In the twenty years following the recognition of the field of nitric oxide by the Nobel Foundation in 1998, many key discoveries made their way from the laboratory setting into our everyday lifestyles. Many of these studies led to a greater understanding of exercise physiology. Others revealed that a variety of food ingredients could promote cardiovascular health and sports performance.

Experimental evidence shows that the best ways to ensure adequate production and action of NO are to adapt a healthy, balanced diet and to engage in frequent physical activity. Without the background knowledge of basic research in nutrition and exercise physiology that we have today, you probably wouldn't believe that all you need to do to prevent Type 2 diabetes, stroke, and heart attack is eat healthy and exercise three to four days a week. You might think if all one needed to do is eat healthy and exercise, why is it that more than 70 percent of the population in the US suffers from one or more forms of cardiovascular disease? The answer is alarmingly straightforward ... as unbelievable as it might seem, the fact is that 70 percent of the US population does NOT follow a healthy lifestyle of eating and exercise. If these people understood how nitric oxide can prevent disease and promote healthy aging, hopefully they would be inspired to make these changes to their lifestyle.

Let's begin first with physical activity or exercise. It's been known for thousands of years that physical activity or exercise is crucial for healthy aging, but the reason for this was unknown until recently. The reason is simple, and it is all about nitric oxide. We've understood, since 2000 or so, that physical activity is vital to providing the nitric oxide that the body requires for healthy aging. Bodily movement stimulates the production of nitric oxide in the endothelial cells lining your arteries. As you exert yourself and move around faster, your heart rate increases, and the blood is pumped through the arteries with more force. This increased force of blood pushing against the vascular endothelial cells signals them to produce more NO. The NO brings about vasodilation and, therefore, increases blood flow. This is important physiologically. All cells, especially muscle cells, need oxygen and nutrients in order to contract and create the force required to move your limbs. Your circulating blood carries oxygen in the red blood cells and nutrients dissolved in the liquid part of the blood, called plasma. Blood circulates near every cell in your body, including the muscle cells. The oxygen and nutrients diffuse from the blood right into the muscle cells. The more strenuous the body movement, such as moderate exercise, the greater the volume of blood that circulates through your arteries (and veins). More blood circulation provides more oxygen and nutrients to the working muscle cells.

But also recall that NO has its own beneficial health effects. NO is produced by our arteries to prevent heart attack, heart failure, and stroke. The NO that is produced in the endothelial cells during physical activity to increase exercise performance and endurance is the very same NO that protects your cardiovascular system against disease. Indeed, it is now well-appreciated that engaging in a regular schedule or program of physical activity throughout your life results in continuous nitric oxide production at a level that is higher than when no exercise is performed. This, in turn, could prevent or lower the risk of heart attack, stroke, diabetes, mental disorders, and many other diseases. Bottom line: good health, exercise, and nitric oxide all go hand-in-hand.

Now let's turn to a healthy balanced diet tied to calorie restriction. Diet is often referred to as a dietary regimen for losing weight. However, diet simply means what food we eat in the course of a day, a week, a month, etc. Being overweight, but not necessarily obese, leads to a decrease in the production and action of NO, which, in turn, often leads to cardiovascular disease.

A balanced diet means eating from all the different food groups in the right quantities. Nutritionists say there are five main food groups to consider: whole grains, fruit and vegetables, protein, dairy, and fat and sugar. There is no merit in focusing on only one or two food groups when the objective is to lose or maintain body weight. Many people are under the false impression that eating mainly protein and cutting out most carbohydrates is the way to lose weight. There is no clinical evidence that such a diet is successful in the long run. In fact, consuming excess protein without carbohydrate balance could lead to problems associated with poor kidney function.

Some foods have a pronounced effect on NO production or action in the body. Saturated fats and table salt (sodium chloride) can markedly interfere with the production of NO by inhibiting the enzyme that produces it. In addition, saturated fats undergo oxidation, forming substances that can quickly destroy NO. Excessive sugar consumption also results in decreased NO production by vascular endothelial cells. Continuous consumption of such foods will result in long-term problems associated with inadequate NO, including Type 2 diabetes, hypertension, atherosclerosis or coronary artery disease, cerebral stroke, and kidney failure. Cutting back on the consumption of such unhealthy foods will go a long way in promoting more NO production and action.

Conversely, increasing your consumption of certain foods will boost your NO production and action. Fish, which contains unsaturated fat and Omega-3 fatty acids, is an excellent example. Avocados and nuts also contain unsaturated fats and Omega-3. Omega-3 fatty acids strengthen the integrity and health of our vascular endothelial cells, thus enabling these cells to produce nitric oxide in a continuous manner. Similarly, fruits and vegetables constitute an essential part of a healthy diet. These foods contain natural antioxidants, which protect NO against oxidative destruction by conditions that create oxidative stress, such as a diet rich in saturated fats, sugar, and salt.

Consuming protein is essential to providing the twenty or so amino acids required by your body to survive. Certain amino acids, including L-arginine and L-citrulline, are required for NO production by vascular endothelial cells and all other cells. Healthy protein sources include fish, nuts, and soybeans. Finally, multigrain foods are essential to consume regularly because they provide fiber and also boost NO levels.

All of these beneficial effects may be attributed, at least in part, to increased production of NO by your vascular endothelial cells. Therefore, vascular integrity and nitric oxide production may be very important in determining healthy aging by virtue of the capacity of NO to normalize blood pressure and prevent inflammation of the arterial wall, thereby curtailing coronary artery disease.

Consumption of beets, which contain nitrate, results in increased production of NO at distant sites in the body. The nitrate serves as a source of NO. But let's not forget about spinach, an iconic symbol of eating healthy mainly thanks to Popeye. Popeye made his comic strip debut in 1929, and his first appearance on film was in a 1933 *Betty Boop* Paramount cartoon called *Popeye the Sailor*. In the comics, Popeye originally derived his great strength from rubbing the head of the Whiffle Hen. By 1932, this gimmick was changed to eating spinach. Spinach not only gave Popeye superhuman strength but also endowed the sailor with abilities like virtuoso dancing or playing piano. The Popeye cartoons were so popular during the Depression that sales of spinach in America increased by 33 percent, and it briefly slotted in as the third most popular kids' food after ice cream and turkey. Imagine that! Kids wanting to eat spinach!

But it wasn't just a cartoon gimmick. The link was made more than fifty years earlier, in 1870, when Erich von Wolf, a German chemist, found that spinach contained more iron than any other leafy green vegetable. Today, we all know that spinach is healthy because of its high iron content. However, it is also equally important to point out that the ingestion of spinach provides a high content of nitrate and nitrite, which are converted to nitric oxide in the body. The nitric oxide indirectly increases strength and exercise endurance by promoting the circulation in your muscles.

As I became more and more convinced that nitric oxide was essential to a healthy lifestyle, I began to pay more attention to my own lifestyle and take the necessary steps to ensure that I always practice what I preach. Moreover, Sharon got on my case to eat healthy and work out more. She could see, as could I, that life as a Nobel Laureate was going to be busy with lots of traveling and eating. It was clear to me that such a change in lifestyle might easily add several inches to my waistline. And so, I adopted a plan to change my eating habits. Sharon and I worked together diligently on this project, and it paid off. We also started to exercise in a systematic manner, running outdoors and working out at a local gymnasium.

We were so motivated by all this exercise that we set a goal to train for the 2004 Los Angeles Marathon. Neither of us had ever run a marathon. After both finishing that unforgiving run, we decided to keep training and run more marathons. We managed to run fourteen more marathons over the next five years.

While chatting with some of the marathon runners in our second marathon, the Chicago marathon, I learned that many of them used iPods to listen to recorded music while they ran. They reported that listening to music was an excellent way of providing a much-needed motivation boost near the end of a 26.2-mile run. And so, when I returned home, I bought an iPod and downloaded dozens of tunes, which I felt could help me maintain my pace during the long runs. Through trial and error, I learned which tunes were best for running. Neither Vivaldi nor Mozart did the trick for me. Baroque classical music was superb for studying and creative writing but not for running marathons. Turns out, it had to be rock music. The Bee Gees, the Beatles, and Elton John were the perfect picks for me.

Elton John's music was the main key to my success in completing most marathons in under four and a half hours. I created my playlist such that Elton John's tunes would play every three miles of running (about every thirty minutes). These tunes included "Someone Saved My Life Tonight," "Daniel," "Rocket Man" and, at mile twenty-one, I programmed my iPod to play "I'm Still Standing" at every mile marker until I crossed the finish line. And, believe me, I was happy to be "Still Standing" after four and a half hours of keeping my heart rate above 120 beats per minute!

Chapter 20:
Full Circle

Although my mother traveled with Sharon and me to Stockholm for the Nobel festivities, and she appeared to be healthy and quite active, a couple of years later, she began to slow down and show signs that living alone was becoming a struggle. Sharon and I entertained the idea of inviting Mom to move in with us, permanently, in Beverly Hills. A priori, knowing how proud and stubborn my mom was, I did not believe she would admit that she was aging enough to vacate her home and move in with us. We decided to wait.

A few short months later, my mom had an alarming accident in her garage that prompted me to take action. As she attempted to retrieve a box that she had stored on a high shelf, the folding step ladder she was standing on gave way and fell. Apparently, Mom had climbed to the very top step, the one that gives a clear warning NOT to stand on it or you could lose your balance. No surprise, she did lose her balance and was left hanging by her hands on a wooden beam ten feet above the ground. Being only five feet tall, this presented a serious problem for her. As her neighbor tells the story, Mom screamed bloody murder for many minutes before he figured out what the screaming was all about. He found her hanging from the beam and successfully took hold of her and safely brought her back down to earth.

I approached Mom and explained that we wanted her to move in with us and that we would take care of the move and also handle the sale of her ranch-style home in Downey, about twenty-five miles from Beverly Hills. At first, Mom hesitated and told us that she was not yet ready to move in with us. She insisted that she was strong and had full control of herself while living alone. Moreover, she reminded us that she still drove her car every day. I reminded her of the incident in her garage and the fact that she could have fallen off the step ladder and crippled herself. Never one to give in to an argument, Mom said that she would never again climb to the top step of the ladder, but she didn't need to leave her home.

Then I struck gold. I said, "Mom, don't you want to live in Beverly Hills? You could tell everyone that you live in Beverly Hills!"

For the first time that I can recall, she paused before responding.

After one minute of silent consideration, Mom asked us which bedroom would become hers. Just as I started to speak, she interrupted me and said loudly, "I'll move in under one condition. I want the biggest bedroom in the house, and with my own bathroom too."

We all agreed that one of the ground-level bedrooms would be best for her so she could avoid having to walk up and down the long staircase to the second-level bedrooms. Still, she wouldn't commit before coming over to our home again to check it out.

When we brought her over to scope out her new digs, Mom was pleased and agreed to the move. So pleased, she asked us if she could move in right away.

I laughed and whispered to Sharon, "One day, she's resisting any such move, and the next day, she wants to move in as soon as possible. That's my mom!"

But I had one condition as well. I said, "After you move in with us, I want you to teach me how to cook all the Italian dishes you used to prepare for the family every Sunday."

"It's about time you asked me! What took you so long?"

About two months after her move to Beverly Hills, Mom informed me that it was time for me to begin cooking.

"Let's go to the supermarket, and I'll show you how to shop." Mom was quite particular in selecting the cuts of meat and the produce, especially eggplant and bell peppers. I asked her a lot of questions, and she said to me, "Don't worry, we're going to do this many more times, and you'll get the hang of it in no time."

After we arrived back home, she told me that we were going to get up early the next morning and begin cooking at 6:00 a.m. sharp. I asked her why we had to start so early, since dinner isn't usually until 6:00 p.m. She said, "Wait, you'll see why."

In preparation for my cooking lessons, I took out a new spiral notebook, and I was all set to take notes. I noted how she cut the beef and pork, which were to be used to prepare the pasta sauce and side dishes. Then things began to get difficult for me. Mom would pour some salt into the palm of one hand and throw it into the pot. She did the same with the pepper. Then she poured olive oil into the pot, without measuring the volume.

"Wait a minute," I interrupted. "How much of everything are you adding? I won't be able to remember all this."

"The amount is not important. Just watch what I do, and next time, you do the same thing."

I already knew that I was never going to be able to reproduce her recipe for meat sauce. But we continued anyway and then went on to prepare the eggplant parmigiana. The first step was to slice the eggplant in a special manner so all pieces were of equal size and thickness. Mom impressed me with her precise surgical skills. I wrote all the details in my cooking notebook. Then, things became difficult once again as she added the salt, pepper, and olive oil without measuring anything. It suddenly dawned on me what I needed to do for the second cooking lesson.

As a scientist, it was imperative that I obtain a more precise means of quantifying the salt, pepper, olive oil, garlic powder, and grated parmesan cheese. "One or two handfuls" was just not going to work for me. I went to my laboratory at UCLA, and I borrowed a scale, some graduated cylinders, and a few beakers. I needed these supplies to make more reproducible measurements of the ingredients. As we began cooking during this second round, and Mom poured salt into her left palm, I stopped her.

"Wait. Put the salt into this container and not into the pot."

"What for? It needs to go in the pot!"

I quickly weighed the salt on my trusty balance and poured it into the pot. We did the same thing with the other ingredients, and I entered the data into my notebook.

"You see, Mom, this is how we do things in the laboratory."

"But this is a kitchen, not a laboratory," Mom said. "You think you know everything! Get outta here!"

Mom and I managed to get through the entire second lesson without much argument. In addition to making meat sauce for the pasta, I could also prepare eggplant parmigiana, although the final product could never win a beauty contest. My best first dish was the thin strips of bell peppers baked in olive oil with capers. My mom, Sharon, and I had dinner that evening, and on the menu was what Mom and I had prepared all day long.

The verdict was fairly good, and Mom said my cooking was, "Good, but not great. You still need to improve."

Personally, I thought it was fabulous. I continued to work with Mom in the kitchen for the next few weeks, and then I asked her if I was ready to cook a special dinner, all by myself, for the entire family on a Sunday afternoon. I was surprised when, without hesitation, Mom said that I was ready.

And so, I organized a date for this special event, which included Mom and Sharon, my brother and his partner, Heather, her husband Jeffrey, my cousin Joey, and a few friends.

This would be a lot of work for me. I divided up the cooking over a two-day period. The meat sauce and the bell pepper dish were prepared the day before and kept cold in the refrigerator. I made the eggplant parmigiana in the morning of the dinner; it took about four hours to prepare this dish alone. The guests arrived at about 2:00 p.m. for a 3:00 p.m. dinner. I poured us all some prosecco, and I called for the guests to drink a toast to Mom, who I told them had worked for two days to prepare this meal for us.

I told no one present that it was actually I who had prepared the entire meal. The words "Salute" and "Cin cin" were shouted repeatedly. We got through the first course of insalata, and everyone loved it. Then out came the rigatoni pasta smothered in the special meat sauce. I've never before heard such moans and groans of pleasure expressed over a delicious dish. The servings of meat, pork, sausage, eggplant, and bell peppers were equally invigorating to the group.

Then came the ultimate compliment. My brother, Angelo, said loudly to the entire group at the table, "Mom, I've been eating your delicious Italian cooking for over forty years, and each and every one has been perfect in every way. But this one is even better yet. It's the best dinner you've ever made. I don't know how you manage to do this time and time again and then actually improve it."

Everyone at the table clapped loudly except Mom and me. Indeed, Mom shouted out, "Get outta here! I didn't cook this meal, not one bit of it—your brother did, and he did it by himself!"

In hearing this, the guests turned their applause to me, though Angelo refused to believe that I cooked any part of the meal. Then Mom jumped in to, once again, take all the credit. She explained how she had spent the last few months working with me and teaching me to cook her style of Italian cuisine. In the end, everyone was pleased, and I gave Mom a big hug and kiss.

Shortly after this momentous occasion, my mom's health started to deteriorate rapidly. She could no longer safely drive her car. She found it increasingly difficult to walk to church on Sundays. Within the following year, she began to lose her balance in the home and took an occasional fall, sometimes quite serious. Sharon and I recognized the need to arrange assisted living for her.

All of this was difficult for me to bear. All my life, I'd remember Mom as being strong, feisty, lively, stubborn, and dominant. When I was a growing child, she always knew what trouble I was up to and took action to set me straight. Whenever I brought home my report card with a grade of A-minus on it, she asked me why not an A. When I raced cars at the drag strip, although she didn't approve, if I were to come in second place, she would ask me why not first place. Although I might not have appreciated it at the time, her setting the bar so high served to motivate me without frustrating me.

All Mom wanted from me was to do the very best I was capable of. I'm certain that she was very proud when I was awarded the Nobel Prize. Moreover, I know she felt she played an important role in my success.

Mom passed on quietly in her sleep in January of 2006, on her ninetieth birthday. I miss her still.

Meeting Elton John

In April of 2005, Herbalife Nutrition celebrated its twenty-fifth anniversary by hosting an extravaganza in Atlanta for about thirty thousand of its top distributors. The event was held in the Georgia Dome, and, since I was on the Scientific Advisory Board of Herbalife, I was invited to participate in the event. The highlight of the gala was a private concert by Elton John.

I was asked if I wished to meet him privately. The arrangement was that I would meet him backstage just prior to his concert. Although I rarely get nervous before I am to meet someone face to face, even a big celebrity, meeting Elton John was different. I paced back and forth for fifteen minutes, trying to calm myself until I heard a voice. "Professor Ignarro, Sir Elton John will see you now!"

My blood pressure rose steadily as I walked over to the short ramp leading up to the back of the stage. The gentleman escorting me up the ramp opened the bright red curtain so I could enter. And there, in front of me, was Elton John. He was dressed in an extravagant, bright-colored Rocket Man costume, wearing extra-thick, wide-rim, yellow glasses. What a sight to see! He was about my height but had much broader shoulders, like a wrestler.

I explained briefly who I was and that I had been awarded the Nobel Prize in Medicine for my work on nitric oxide and cardiovascular health. He quickly interjected, "Yes, I know who you are, and I congratulate you." But the ultimate surprise and compliment came when he asked if I was the person who invented Viagra.

"Sort of," I told him, and I explained how my research made possible the invention of the little blue pill by a large pharmaceutical company.

Elton was very much interested in how Viagra was developed and asked me to explain exactly what my role was in the development of this blockbuster drug.

Accordingly, in layman's terms, I explained how I discovered nitric oxide and the role I played in creating Viagra.

Elton said, "Hum," and paused for a moment. Then, he asked me a truly provocative question. "What about men with normal erectile function? Would they benefit from taking Viagra?"

"There's only one way to find out, right?"

He laughed out loud, which nearly startled me because his voice really carries.

Elton continued by asking me if I had ever taken any Viagra.

This time, I paused for a moment and then said, "Elton, I'm Italian; I don't have to take any Viagra!"

Once again, he laughed loudly and said, "Very good, Professor Ignarro."

Elton then asked me what year I was awarded the Nobel Prize. I told him that my lucky year was 1998. Without hesitation, I said to him, "1998 was a very good year. Weren't you knighted by the Queen of England in 1998?"

"Yes!" he responded. He was so impressed that I recalled the year that he had been knighted. After my comment, he immediately asked me for my autograph.

Imagine that. Elton John asked Lou Ignarro for his autograph!

He then asked, "Are you familiar with my music?"

"What, are you kidding me?" I said. "I'm familiar with every single one of your songs!"

"Name your three favorites," he said.

"'I'm Still Standing,' 'Crocodile Rock,' and 'Sacrifice,'" I said. I then went on to explain the special significance of "I'm Still Standing" during my marathon runs.

Elton was summoned to get ready for his performance.

He gave me a big hug and said it was a delight to meet me.

I told him the honor and pleasure were all mine.

As he walked away, one of his staff escorted me to my seat in the concert hall, in the front row about ten feet from the stage, directly in front of Elton's piano. Elton John's performance was brilliant, colorful, and full of energy. He sang most of his top hits during the ninety-minute concert, and each one sounded as professional and polished as his original recordings, which is a testament to his perfection as a musician and performer. The colorful light show on stage was matched only by his extraordinary clothes and shoes. One highlight of his performance was when he completed a song, ran to the back of the piano, and jumped and slid along the top of the piano toward the audience, landing upright on the edge of the stage. I thought, for a moment, that his momentum would carry him off the stage into my lap. But he caught himself just in time.

Near the end of the concert, staring directly at me, Elton John told the audience that he wanted to play three tunes at the request of Professor Lou Ignarro. His final song was "I'm Still Standing."

As Christmas day was rapidly approaching, instead of doing our routine morning runs, we decided to relax in the living room near the Christmas tree. Sharon recalled that she had an old Lionel train set stored in a box in the attic. It had belonged to her dad. She told me it was about seventy years old and asked me if we could set it up and run it around the Christmas tree. *Great idea*, I thought. And so, I examined the train set and cleaned and lubricated the critical parts. It operated fairly well. As I sat on the sofa, watching that Lionel train chug along the tracks, something hit me. The memories of my own Lionel train layout many years prior flashed before my eyes. I got the urge to build a new model railroad. I asked Sharon if she would accompany me to a local model railroad store to look at some trains.

She knew exactly what I had in mind, and she agreed. We looked at quite a few train sets, locomotives, freight cars, passenger cars, and accessories. I could not get over all of the advances made in this hobby over the sixty years since I'd last shopped for a train set. One could now operate the trains and accessories by remote control and program the locomotives to move around the layout according to predetermined scenarios. The trains were realistic in appearance, detail, and sounds. I couldn't resist any longer. I bought a set, took it home, and put it up around the Christmas tree near the existing 1950s train set.

When the Christmas season came to a close and we had to take down the tree, Sharon asked me what I was going to do with the new train set I had just purchased. I told her that I'd like to keep it on the floor in a corner of the living room just for a few more weeks. She agreed, as long as I didn't scratch the wooden floors. During the next few weeks, I enjoyed building a nice layout with realistic scenery, buildings, cars, and people figures. I even purchased a second train set for the layout. At about this time, we had already decided to undergo a major remodel of our home in Beverly Hills. Included in our plans was a garage rebuild, since it was in such bad shape that we had to park our cars in the driveway. Then, I entertained the thought of using the new garage for parking my train layout instead of the cars. Much to my surprise and delight, Sharon agreed. She was also in favor of my idea of building a larger garage for the layout.

Several months later, construction complete, I initiated what turned out to be a five-year project to build the train layout of my dreams. I did every stitch of the work myself, including the carpentry, electrical wiring, scenery, bridges, lighting, and individual scenes. All of the materials and trains were purchased from The Train Shack located in Burbank, California. The owners of the shop were favorably impressed with my layout and arranged for a prominent national train magazine (*O-Gauge Railroading*) to visit my home and shoot videos of my layout for publication.

Linus Pauling

In 2019, I was invited to the Linus Pauling Institute (LPI) at Oregon State University in Corvallis to give a public Nobel lecture about the role of nitric oxide in healthy lifestyle and longevity. I cannot recall being more excited about a speaking invitation than this one. Linus Pauling had been the first Nobel Laureate I'd met, way back when I was only a fifteen-year-old high school student. I had never forgotten his visit and the motivating influence he had on my development as a student and scientist. And now, I was going to his institute to speak as an invited Nobel Laureate. It just doesn't get much better than that!

In 1973, Pauling co-founded the LPI, which was established primarily to conduct research and education in orthomolecular medicine, following his belief that nutritional supplementation could prevent, ameliorate, or cure many diseases, slow the aging process, and alleviate suffering. At the LPI, Pauling and his coworkers researched developing diagnostic tests and tools for analyzing a multitude of compounds found in body fluids.

Pauling's insights were ahead of his time. He believed that biochemical individuality, involving unique dietary needs specific to individuals, determines how optimum health can be achieved through the judicious use of natural substances or nutritional supplements. He maintained that biochemical individuality, such as existing disease or stress, could increase the need for certain micronutrients, such as vitamin C. Pauling also warned against overconsumption of potentially unhealthy substances such as sugar and chemical sweeteners. He considered orthomolecular or nutritional medicine as a crucial adjunct to standard medical practice and, therefore, did not rule out conventional treatments such as surgery, radiation, chemotherapy, and other drugs to treat existing disease.

As a prominent, knowledgeable, and articulate spokesman for the use of nutritional supplements as a means to achieve a healthy lifestyle, Pauling gained a large number of ardent admirers among the public. He also had doubters and detractors, but Pauling's scientific evidence was convincing, and many investigators went on to confirm and strengthen his beliefs. He utilized the media's ongoing interest in him to good effect in promoting his "regimen for better health," with vitamin C as its cornerstone.

Today, the investigators at the LPI have a focused interest in nutritional medicine and the mechanism of action of many naturally occurring substances. Linus Pauling was considered by his peers to be a master at explaining difficult, even abstruse, medical and scientific information in terms that were understandable to intelligent laypersons. I can attest to that, having spoken with Pauling when he visited my high school back in 1956. He had the ability to explain chemical principles in a way that stuck in my mind. His explanations were always linked to examples in nature or personal experiences, which made it easier to remember and recall later on.

I was about to give my special talk, termed the public lecture, in a large auditorium on campus. The audience consisted of community citizens plus students and faculty at the LPI. In addition, faculty from the University of Oregon in nearby Eugene were invited to attend my lecture and chat with me at the reception to follow. As I usually do before I speak, I walked into the auditorium about a half-hour early to relax and familiarize myself with the stage and tools. This also gave me the opportunity to watch the crowd gradually walk into the auditorium and take their seats. I personally welcomed many of the attendees and thanked them for coming to my talk. The expressions on their faces were always worth my efforts, as some looked surprised that I would come over to say hello to them. Doing this also gave me lots of familiar faces to look at while speaking so I did not feel that I was speaking to a bunch of total strangers.

I deliberately focused my lecture on Linus Pauling's long-standing theme of advocating proper nutrition to prevent disease and foster healthy living. This was easy for me because, like Pauling, I've been a long-standing advocate of healthy nutrition for healthy aging. Accordingly, I spoke about the role of nitric oxide in a healthy lifestyle and longevity. Undoubtedly, if Pauling had been alive to hear my speech, he would have been pleased with the extensive, modern basic research demonstrating that many natural substances such as antioxidants, certain vitamins, amino acids, and proteins all promote the production and action of NO, which is essential for health and longevity.

Midway through my talk, I explained that, in my research experiments, I had used vitamin C as an antioxidant to stabilize EDRF so we could then isolate and identify it as nitric oxide. Upon hearing that, the audience cheered and applauded, likely because they were familiar with the world-famous research on vitamin C by Linus Pauling. I followed this by explaining that one of the most important health benefits of vitamin C is increasing your levels of nitric oxide by delaying its breakdown in the body.

As I proceeded with my talk, I felt more and more comfortable and in tune with the audience, who was paying close attention to what I was teaching. Moreover, I felt as close as ever to

Linus Pauling. Here I was in the auditorium of the Linus Pauling Institute, giving a public lecture in his name. As I continued speaking, I recalled my brief, yet unforgettable encounter with Pauling when I was a boy in high school who happened to be curious about chemistry. I felt as if Linus Pauling were sitting right there in the audience, and it gave me the sense that, at least in some small way, he'd been with me all along.

THE END

Epilogue

New discoveries pertaining to the biological actions of nitric oxide never seem to end. Experimental and clinical evidence indicates that nitric oxide is effective in the treatment of COVID-19 brought on by the SARS CoV-2 virus. NO has been well known to help fight infection. Your body's defense against invading microorganisms such as bacteria, viruses, protozoa, and fungi is mediated in large part by nitric oxide.

Many types of viruses are inhaled into the lungs and can cause pulmonary and systemic inflammation and infection, leading to pneumonia and worse. In addition to viruses that cause influenza, some can bring about far more serious pulmonary disease. One prime example is SARS CoV-2, the coronavirus that causes COVID-19. This virus must enter the lungs by inhalation to be harmful to the host. The coronavirus attaches to cells deep inside the lungs and begins to replicate and spread. The single most important target for the coronavirus is the arterial endothelial cell layer, which lines every blood vessel in the lungs. The coronavirus attacks the endothelial cells, causing an inflammatory response that kills these cells. Since the endothelial cells are responsible for all the nitric oxide produced by blood vessels, NO production in the lungs decreases dramatically.

The NO produced by these cells is required to keep the arteries dilated so the oxygen-containing blood can flow through. Moreover, NO prevents the blood from clotting in the lungs. In COVID-19, the depletion of NO results in pulmonary hypertension, inadequate oxygen delivery, and massive blood coagulation or thrombosis, which ultimately kills the host by suffocation. The depleted endothelium-derived NO can be easily replaced by inhalation of commercially available NO gas. Recent clinical trials have demonstrated that inhaled NO therapy is effective in treating COVID-19 patients by reversing the inflammation and thrombosis brought about by a deficiency in NO.

Administering inhaled NO gas to patients with COVID-19 could provide an important adjunct in the treatment of this potentially fatal disease. If patients with early stages of COVID-19 receive NO, the resulting beneficial therapeutic effects might keep them from having to be admitted to the ICU. This would free up rooms, beds, and oxygen for those who require them to stay alive. Inhaled NO could offer great benefits during this pandemic, which does not appear to be ending anytime soon. The effectiveness of NO in treating patients with COVID-19 has already motivated many biotech companies to manufacture handheld devices for the safe self-administration of NO by inhalation. Such devices should be available soon but would need to be approved by the FDA before they can be made widely available to the public. Assuming such approval, this therapeutic method could be used outside the hospital or clinic, providing safe, easy, and effective care right from the comfort of your own home.

Acknowledgements

I was inspired to write this book by my wife, Sharon, and my brother, Angelo, who both believed that my life story and climb to success were so different from most individuals and needed to be told. As I contemplated embarking on such a monumental project, I received feedback from my former students, postdoctoral fellows, and many collaborating scientists, all of whom jumped on the bandwagon to get me to write this memoir. Finally, I gave in and started writing. At the very start, I made a chronological outline of what memorable events I might want to put in my book. When I completed this task, about four months later, I realized for the first time that this just might be a damn good book. And so, I began to take a more serious approach to my writing.

Shortly into my assignment, however, I came to the realization that I did not know how to write. I started writing my book as if I were writing one of my scientific articles, and boy was it boring. I became depressed and concluded that I could never write a book that would interest the lay public. But then, my friend and colleague, Dr. Will Li from Boston, saved the day. Will strongly recommended that I contact a highly experienced and successful writing coach to help me out. I jumped at the opportunity and hired Ms. Robin Colucci, who was residing in Connecticut. She said to me "Lou, why don't you send me the manuscript of what you have thus far, and then I'll make a decision." So, I did just that and waited for her response. We communicated by Zoom calls. On our first call, I thought she might say that my writing was not her cup of tea, and she would pass on this project. Instead, she really liked what I had written and said we just had to modify it a bit. I followed up with "just what is a bit," and she said "actually, a lot."

As I thrive on pressure and hard work, I signed a contract with Robin, which was the most important thing I've done regarding my book. She did not write a single word for me. Instead, she coached me relentlessly, reorganized my brain and way of thinking, and suggested a different kind of writing style. Miraculously, she showed me how to transform my incredibly boring prose into exciting conversation involving the creation of exciting scenes. After a while, I got so good at it that she had to slow me down, informing me that I was not writing a screenplay. If my book, *Dr. NO*, turns out to be successful, I owe it all to Robin Colucci. Thanks Robin.

Very importantly, major thanks and credit must be given to all past members of the Ignarro Laboratory who created the Nobel Prize-earning body of work described in this book. They are way too numerous to mention here because of space restrictions, but you know who you are. Many of the active players are described over and over again in this book. Throughout my basic research career, I had the good fortune and opportunity to work with many of the best scientists in the world. Each and every one of them gave me the critical assistance I needed during each step of my path to success. And, as fate would have it, each of them went on to be awarded the Nobel Prize. These individuals include Linus Pauling, Julius Axelrod, Christian De Duve, Paul Greengard, Andrew Schally, and Sir John Vane.

I want to give thanks to the three institutions in which I had productive research programs, including Ciba Geigy Pharmaceuticals (later called Novartis), Tulane University Medical Center, and UCLA. Thanks to the National Institutes of Health (NIH) for funding nearly all of my basic research that led to the Nobel Prize. Without such government funding, I would not be writing this book.

Finally, special thanks go to Richard Joseph and Vertel Publishing for believing in the concept of Dr. NO from the beginning, and sticking with it until completion.